FOOT THERAPY FOR CHILDREN

A textbook concerned primarily with the pre-natal, natal and postnatal problems of the feet and the lower extremities in infancy and childhood.

BY

Philip R. Brachman, A.B.; D.S.C.

Chairman Department of Orthopedics Illinois College of Podiatry. Professor of Podopediatrics Illinois College of Podiatry. Chief of Podiatry Surgical Staff American Hospital. Chief of Podiatry Section Beef Bone Cutters and Sausage Makers Union Clinic. Consultant in Podiatry Chicago Rehabilitation Institute. Consultant in Podiatry Mercy Hospital. Consultant Shoe Service Institute.

Podiatry Books Co.
18 South Michigan Ave.
Chicago, Ill.

Printed by Interstate Printers and Publishers
Danville, Illinois.
U.S.A.

PREFACE

Twenty five years ago I organized my first lecture course dealing with foot problems in children. This textbook is the culmination of that lecture course. There is no attempt made in these pages to offer the comprehensive diagnosis, care and treatment of all problems related to the foot and lower extremity of the infant and the young child. I would much rather describe this book as a personal approach to the problem during the past twenty five years and then express the hope that some of my former students and colleagues will fill in the gaps in the future.

As do all men who fulfill the urge to write textbooks, I owe more than I can ever repay to all who have taught me through the written and spoken word. If I have succeeded somewhat in my efforts it was because of those who have left us their great legacy of medical and scientific knowledge.

However, I have also been most fortunate in help that I have received over the years from my associates in Medicine and Podiatry. Joseph L. Koczur, M.D.; more than any other has been most helpful and most inspiring. When I first started to work with children Robert T. McElvenny, M.D.; directed some of my early efforts and I will never forget his unselfish help. At a later date I received much from my association with Robert Addison, M.D. and Allen Hirschtick, M.D.

Peter M. Varzos, with whom I have been associated for the past twenty years has worked with me to develop many of the thoughts and methods of care reported in this book and I owe him much for his efforts. Above all others my thanks must go to my wife Jane for her help and devotion to the arduous task of compiling this book and making it become a reality.

Finally I want to thank Wade Liggett for his professional proof reading efforts, Howard Moore for all of his good services and all of the members of his staff for their help. My thanks also go to the administrations of those Podiatry Colleges who had enough faith in my efforts to use this book as a teaching text for their classes and to the personnel of The Interstate Printers and Publishers, Inc., who put up with me during the publishing of this book.

CONTENTS

INTRODUCTION
TO PODOPEDIATRICS

Podopediatrics is that phase of podiatry which deals with infants and children. It is our contention that a podiatrist must understand the foot of the infant and child and must have a clear concept of the embryology of the foot before he can give adequate treatment to the adult patients. In the treatment of infants and children, the podiatrist does not deal with a foot of an infant or child but with an infant or child who has a foot problem. While in essence these foot problems may be quite similar to those of the adults, there are many factors attending them that we do not see in the adult. For purposes of convenience, most of the problems attending infants may be divided into prenatal, natal and postnatal classifications.

Prenatal Problems

In the prenatal group, we must consider such difficulties as cerebral palsy and other injuries affecting the brain, the spinal cord, and many orthopedic lesions of the feet including clubfoot and the more rare problems affecting the circulatory system, the glandular system, and the integument of the body. Some of these will be dealt with individually in succeeding pages.

Natal Problems

The many injuries which attend the actual birth of the child may also have a considerable amount of influence on foot pathology. In the main, these are associated with injuries of the neurological system which may be caused by lack of oxygen, a deficiency in the blood supply, or trauma.

Postnatal Problems

In the consideration of postnatal injuries we must concern ourselves primarily with those factors that attend the life of the child for the first three months. Here again we must consider constitutional difficulties that may affect any child, injuries which may occur to the child outside of its protective environment in utero, problems of digestion, food and chemical poisonings and a host of other factors. Young infants are immune to a number of diseases and disease organisms, yet there are some organisms which take their heavy toll during infancy. As the infant begins to sit up, crawl, stand, walk and run about, the factors which may cause foot problems increase rapidly.

Footgear

For many millions of years man did not concern himself about footgear. It has only been about two thousand years that shoes have presented another hazard to the foot. During the rise of our so-called civilization, most children have not been hampered by the use of footgear until the past several hundred years. Thus, we see that footgear has not played a part in the evolutionary development of the human foot. Shoes can cause trouble to the foot of the infant if the shoes are not fitted properly, however, most shoe manufacturers today produce shoes that are very adequate for children.

Podiatrists realize that mothers in the United States are greatly concerned over shoes for their infants and children. This concern has become more and more evident in recent years in proportion to the advertising claims of the manufacturers representing this shoe or that shoe as possessing health features. Shoes do not have therapeutic value for infants and children as well as adults. At best, shoes are only a protective covering for the foot; at worst, they can produce a considerable amount of injury if they are not fitted properly or if they are not constructed from the proper materials. However, shoes may be used as a housing for corrective measures whenever the foot requires such measures.

Musculoskeletal

The development of musculoskeletal deformities in children, especially the development of those deformities in the feet, may be slow and insidious. Bennet suggests that at the inception of these deformities there is no specific pain, swelling, fever or unconsciousness or other signs commonly associated with impending disaster, and so the physician does not consider its appearance of primary importance. By the time the physician finally realizes that all is not well, deformities are far advanced and largely uncorrectable.

Neurological

We contend that most foot deformities that are associated with neurological problems, such as those we find in brain-injured children or in children with spina bifida and those foot deformities that are associated with problems of genetic origin, are not difficult to diagnose and invariably receive immediate attention. Problems which are associated with a faulty posture or a faulty position, where the etiology is vague or uncertain, can very often prove far more stubborn than the more obvious deformities. These problems will develop in direct proportion to the intrinsic strength of the tissues involved and the forces of the stresses applied to the tissues together with a period of time that the stresses are applied.

It is important for us to realize that we can brook no compromise in the treatment of these deformities. It is never enough for us to assume that because there is some correction we can stop treatment. Everything possible must be done for these children's foot problems until we arrive at the point of complete correction and until we have assured ourselves that deformities are not likely to occur in the near future. The modalities for corrections are many and varied and we will take them up as we discuss the individual foot problems.

We must point out here that deformities of the feet develop more rapidly than deformities of most other parts of the body because of the highly specialized function of the feet, and these deformities may become irreversible if they do not receive immediate attention. The fact that such deformities are not associated with impending disaster does not permit the parents, the doctors and all others associated with the care of these deformities to neglect them as disgracefully as they have been all these years. The relationship between foot deformities, the deformities of the knees, hips and spine and other severe manifestations of disease entities of the body, including those of the viscera, has never been properly documented. Some future investigators may well berate us for our negligent attitude toward foot deformities in the past.

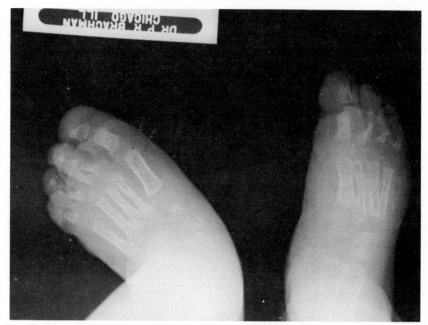

Fig. 1. Bone Structure in Female Spina Bifida, Age Two—Non Ambulatory.

Complexity of the Foot

There is no other single organ of the body whose structure is as complex as that of the infant foot. The embryological development of the foot makes a very fascinating study. Investigators have found that they cannot research the human foot as they have the heart, kidneys and other specialized organs of the human body because of the maze of problems they are led into once they begin their investigations. At the present time there is disagreement between investigators on the physiology of the foot. Every year new concepts are developed and old concepts are revived. At the present time, we have no true authority on foot function and no one has mastered the many problems that are associated with ailing feet.

It may well be that no one will ever be able to study the foot as a single entity because it is too closely associated with the vascular, neurological, glandular, and other systemic activities of the body. But those of us who devote our lives to the care and treatment of the human foot must do everything possible to record even the smallest findings which

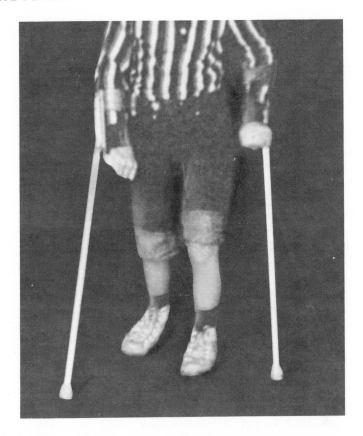

Fig. 2. Six Year Old Male—Spina Bifida—Walks with Special Canes—Wears Keds with Roberts Plates to Support Flail Ankles.

will help our patients in the rehabilitation of the foot. We cannot wait for great discoveries which may never come. It is interesting to note that while research animals can be used in the investigation of problems relating to most organs of the human body, there is no single animal whose foot approaches that of man, and we are therefore extremely limited in the use of research facilities.

Uterogestation and Exterogestation

Montigue writes, "Why are human beings born in a state so immature that it takes eight to ten months before the human infant can even crawl and another four to six months before he can walk and talk?

That a good many years will elapse before the human child will cease to depend upon others for his very survival constitutes yet another evidence of the fact that man is born and remains more immature for a longer period than any other animal."

Man is usually classified with those animals who have a long gestation period such as the elephant with 670 days, the fallow deer with 230 days and the seal whose period varies from 245 to 350 days and yet the newborn young of these three animals are active immediately after birth. In fact, the seal breaks away from his mother at six weeks of age and navigates the waters for himself. It is quite clear that these animals are born and become ready to take care of themselves within a short period after birth but man is the exception to this rule. The theory is proposed by Dr. Montigue that the size of man's brain has increased so much since he developed the upright position that the head, which includes the brain, increased accordingly in size and if he weren't born when he is he wouldn't be born at all.

The average volume of the human brain at birth is 350 cc. By the end of the first year the average volume is 800 cc's which means that about two-thirds of the total growth of the brain is achieved by the end of the first year. Since the average volume of the human brain is 1250 cc's and that growth is attained by most children at four years of age, it can be readily seen how important it is to have the child born when his brain is no more than 350 cc's because if it were any larger it would never pass through the birth canal.

In other words, our children must be born by nine months of age or they cannot be born at all and they require the additional time for the growth of the head to be developed outside of the womb which we call exterogestation. Thus we see that all infants are born prematurely, if we would follow this thesis, and they all need a great deal of attention until they are able to walk.

Growth and Development

It is known that the unborn infant learns to breathe, kick, move around, cough and swallow in utero. That is why babies born prematurely in the seventh month can perform as they do. However, birth marks a new state in the life history of Homo sapiens and requires major adjustments, some of which take two to three weeks for completion. There is the establishment of a normal breathing rhythm, changes in the heart and circulation, adjustment to temperatures of the world outside of the mother, and changes in the method of nutrition must be learned. While most normal children are born with internal resources to overcome these adjustments, these are still challenges. Indeed, a full-term infant is still anatomically and physiologically immature.

General Factors of Growth and Development

A. Problems of nutrition, education and mental health.

B. Processes and stages of growth and development is necessary for effective management of children's health.

C. Recognition of normal variations occurring among children is important—within the limits of the general human pattern—influenced by heredity and environment.

How a Child Differs from an Adult

Body proportions: The head of the child is twenty-five per cent of the body length while the head of the adult is ten per cent of his total body length. A child increases rapidly in size compared to an adult. The average infant's birth weight is tripled at one year of age and the one year weight is doubled at five years, while the five-year weight is tripled by ten years. The length of an infant at one year is one to one and one-half times that at birth and is doubled by the fourth year, tripled by the thirteenth or fourteenth year.

There is a marked variation in the relation of diseases that affect the child and the adult. Infectious diseases produce a very high fever in infants; these infants can appear quite sick but symptoms subside rapidly. The adult could never overcome such high fevers and the adult's symptoms do not subside as rapidly as those of the infant. The need for fluids and minerals during illness is very great in children and infants, but not quite as important in adults. When a child becomes ill and diarrhea develops the illness may become critical after a few hours as the child is dehydrated quickly and reaches a state of acidosis.

Infants and children are suceptible to certain diseases. These include the basic functional diseases related to breathing, metabolism of infants, the effect of congenital malformations of the heart, the palate and the bones, to infants who are immune to measles and diphtheria, and to infants who are prone to otitis media. In early childhood there is much more susceptibility to common contagious diseases, particularly during the school years. During the adolescent period problems relate to growth, development and emotional changes. Finally, children are susceptible to nutritional diseases and to chronic diseases such as tuberculosis and diseases of the neuromuscular system.

Factors Relating to the Growth and Development of the Infant and Young Child

The sense of taste and smell is present at birth and becomes very acute in a short time. It is natural for the child to put things into its mouth until it is two years of age. If this tendency is continued later, the child may be mentally deficient. The infant can distinguish light from darkness and follow a bright object. At five or six months he cries when unfamiliar people come near him. Hearing is acute in the infant a few days after birth. Soothing noises please the infant at four months of age. The development of speech is a measure of intellectual progress.

Emotional development is an orderly process. The mother is the most important factor in the behavior pattern of a healthy child. A child begins to develop independent attitudes at two years of age and completes them after adolescence. These attitudes are not to be hurried or retarded but must be properly directed.

Intellectual Growth

Intelligence is the ability to learn from experience. There are two types of intelligence and both are determined congenitally. The first is formal intelligence which is associated with formal learning and is measurable. The second is contentional and is related to common sense and shrewdness. Intellectual capacity remains constant over a period of years unless interference occurs as a result of disease or injury.

Behavior and Basic Drives

The desire for food and the desire for love and affection are found in all children regardless of any problem that might bring them to your office and these drives must be fulfilled by the parents. As the child gets older, society places barriers on these drives as it necessarily must. Nevertheless, these drives are essential for the emotional development of a child but require modification for acceptance by society.

Foot and Superstructure

The question is often asked, "How does the podiatrist justify his position when he thinks in terms of knee problems, hip problems, and back problems, or when he thinks in terms of systemic diseases as related to local manifestations?" It might also be asked, "Why does the podiatrist study for six years when all he does is take care of the foot problems per se?" The answer to this question is relatively simple. While there is no delineation between the structures such as the nerves, blood vessels, veins, tendons, ligaments, lymph channels, and other structures that enter the foot and are related to the total well-being of the rest of the body, topographically the foot can be described as an entity which can be treated locally, just as the eye can be treated locally or as the nose or ear or mouth can be treated locally.

However, there is no denying the fact that the foot is related to many other tissues and other structures, and that it is associated with and attacked by many diseases that may manifest themselves in other parts of the body.

How, then, does the podiatrist relate himself to these problems? It is the philosophy of the podiatrist that he is educated for and capable of taking care of all problems related to the foot. However, if those problems have systemic manifestations, he is well enough schooled in these manifestations to make it his duty to call in consultants when systemic problems do occur in relationship to foot conditions. Thus, if a patient is diabetic, he will not treat the diabetes per se but he will take care of all foot problems that are related to the disease and call for the family doctor or the internist to take care of the diabetes.

Again, where mechanical problems are concerned and a child walks with a marked pigeon-toed gait, as a result of limitation of external rotation at the hips, he is dealing with a foot problem which produces a pathological gait and will certainly interfere with that patient's ability to walk normally and to grow up with healthy feet if the in-toeing persists and no treatment is available. Here again, the treatment is directed to the feet and carried out with devices that are directly associated with foot function, even though the indirect result will be to stretch the capsules and the ligaments with all other related structures at the hip joint.

Without full knowledge and comprehension of the problems that exist in the superstructure, it would be impossible for the podiatrist to do his work properly. Furthermore, the podiatrist is trained to fully understand all systemic problems which may arise in the hip joint, such as tuberculosis, rheumatoid arthritis, osteochondritis, slipped femoral epiphysis, and hip dysplasia. He has made a thorough study of the anatomy of the hip, the function of the hip, and the treatment of all conditions that may exist in hip-related structures. He is also taught that all problems not related to mechanical gait deficiencies must be referred to a medical specialist whenever the diagnosis seems to point in that direction.

Many anxious parents bring their children to the podiatrist when they find the child is limping or not walking properly because they do not know what is ailing the child, and in a great many instances the

podiatrist is the first professional man to see the child with these difficulties. We feel it is very important for him to have a full knowledge
of these problems so that he may cooperate more closely with the parents
and any member of the medical team called on for consultation. It
would be truly unfortunate if the podiatrist did not understand these
problems and consequently not able to cooperate fully with his medical
colleagues.

2. SCHOOLS FOR PHYSICALLY HANDICAPPED CHILDREN

The physically handicapped children always present a most significant problem in every community. The Chicago Public Schools, under the direction of Dr. Margaret Hall Powers, developed a diagnostic classification of children in special schools for the physically handicapped and for home teaching. This diagnostic category may be of some significance here. In a total of 1,372 children in four elementary and one high school where these children attend classes daily, the breakdown in percentages and diagnostic categories may be seen in the adjoining table. It will be noted particularly that the cerebral palsy children, numbering 464, make up 33.8% of this total volume of handicapped children. The second significant figures are those who have poliomyelitis; this includes 298 children or 21.7% of all children attending these schools. The third largest category are the cardiacs with ninety children or 6.6%, followed by congenital defects and disabilities with eighty-five children or 6.2%, and muscular dystrophy with sixty-five children or 4.7%; the diagnosis of idiopathic sclerosis includes fifty-six children, with 4.1% and spina bifida with forty-three children or 3.1%. Even though poliomyelitis has not been a prominent factor in crippling as many children as it used to, the larger communities have an influx of children from rural areas who are still affected from this crippling disease, as is evidenced by the large number still attending these schools. It may be interesting to repeat some of the random notes taken during a clinical session held at one of the schools where ten of the children were seen, all with foot problems.

11

DIAGNOSTIC CLASSIFICATION OF CHILDREN IN SPECIAL SCHOOLS FOR PHYSICALLY HANDICAPPED AND ON HOME INSTRUCTION CHICAGO PUBLIC SCHOOLS

Prepared by Margaret Hall Powers, Director
Bureau of Physically Handicapped Children and Division of Speech Correction

November, 1965

Diagnostic Category	Homebound		SPECIAL SCHOOLS													
			Burbank		Christopher		Neil		Spalding* Elementary		Total Elementary		Spalding* High School		Total All Schools	
	No.	%	No.	%	No.	%	No.	%	No.	%	No.	%	No.	%	No.	%
Cerebral Palsy	7	4.2	96	57.5	87	36.1	60	33.0	164	34.0	407	37.9	116	32.0	523	36.4
Poliomyelitis	7	4.2	6	3.6	43	17.8	29	15.9	105	21.7	183	17.1	83	22.9	266	18.5
Cardiac	11	6.6	7	4.2	8	3.3	6	3.3	18	3.7	39	3.6	11	3.0	50	3.5
Congenital defects and disabilities	17	10.2	14	8.4	15	6.2	17	9.3	38	7.9	84	7.8	18	5.0	102	7.1
Muscular Dystrophy	9	5.4	10	6.0	12	5.0	15	8.2	26	5.4	63	5.9	12	3.3	75	5.2
Spina Bifida	1	.6	13	7.8	7	2.9	7	3.8	10	2.1	37	3.4	14	3.9	51	3.6
T.B. bone and joint					1	.4	1	.5			2	.2	2	.6	4	.3
Legg-Perthes disease	8	4.8	5	3.0	7	2.9	7	3.8	11	2.3	30	2.8			30	2.1
Slipped epiphysis	13	7.8			5	2.1	2	1.1	6	1.2	13	1.2	27	7.5	40	2.8
Hemophilia	1	.6	1	.6	14	5.8	2	1.1	9	1.9	26	2.4	5	1.4	31	2.2
Arthritis	3	1.8	2	1.2	1	.4	2	1.1	4	.8	7	.7	8	2.2	15	1.0
Amputation (non-congenital)					5	2.1	2	1.1	4	.8	11	1.0	2	.6	13	.9
Asthma			1	.6	4	1.7	5	2.7	6	1.2	16	1.5	3	.8	19	1.3

(Continued on next page)

November, 1965

SPECIAL SCHOOLS

Diagnostic Category	Homebound No.	%	Burbank No.	%	Christopher No.	%	Neil No.	%	Spalding* Elementary No.	%	Total Elementary No.	%	Spalding* High School No.	%	Total All Schools No.	%
Brain pathology (miscellaneous conditions)	3	1.8			6	2.5	2	1.1	21	4.3	29	2.7	6	1.7	35	2.4
Epilepsy (without other disability)	2	1.2			4	1.7	1	.5			5	.4	3	.8	8	.6
Fracture and non-congenital dislocation	55	33.1			4	1.7	2	1.1	8	1.7	14	1.3	8	2.2	22	1.5
Friedreich's ataxia	9	5.4							3	.6	3	.3	3	.8	6	.4
Nephritis or nephrosis	1	.6			1	.4	2	1.1	3	.6	6	.6	3	.8	9	.6
Osteogenesis imperfecta	1	.6	1	.6	2	.8	2	1.1	2	.4	7	.7	5	1.4	12	.8
Osteomyelitis	1	.6	1	.6					5	1.0	6	.6	2	.6	8	.6
Sickle Cell anemia					2	.8	6	3.3	3	.6	11	1.0	3	.8	14	1.0
Traumatic injuries (excluding fractures)	2	1.2	3	1.8	6	2.5	2	1.1	8	1.7	19	1.8	4	1.1	23	1.6
Tumor (excluding brain tumor)	3	1.8	1	.6	2	.8	2	1.1	1	.2	6	.6	2	.6	8	.6
Miscellaneous (Scoliosis)	12	7.2	6	3.6	5	2.1	10	5.5	28	5.8	49	4.6	22	6.1	71	4.9
TOTAL SCHOOL MEMBERSHIP	166	99.7	167	100.1	241	100.0	182	99.7	483	99.9	1073	100.1	362	100.1	1435	99.9

* Excluding blind and brain injured without other disability.

DISABILITY TRENDS—1954 to 1965
CHILDREN IN SPECIAL SCHOOLS FOR PHYSICALLY HANDICAPPED
CHICAGO PUBLIC SCHOOLS

Prepared by Margaret Hall Powers, Ph.D., Director
Bureau of Physically Handicapped Children and Division of Speech Correction

Diagnostic* Category	April 1954		Dec. 1956		Nov. 1958		Nov. 1959		Nov. 1960		Nov. 1961		Nov. 1962		Nov. 1963		Nov. 1964		Nov. 1965	
	No.	%	No.	%	No.	%	No.	%	No.	%	No.	%	No.	%	No.	%	No.	%	No.	%
Cerebral Palsy	448	33.3	447	32.3	445	32.0	427	31.3	431	32.0	427	32.2	476	35.1	476	34.7	477	34.7	523	36.4
Poliomyelitis	291	21.6	301	21.8	335	24.1	340	24.9	326	24.2	331	25.0	316	23.3	292	21.3	265	19.3	266	18.5
Congenital defects: Excluding spina bifida	74	5.6	62	4.4	109	7.8	91	6.7	81	6.0	89	6.7	90	6.6	90	6.6	82	6.0	102	7.1
Spina Bifida	36	2.7	35	2.6	44	3.2	43	3.2	42	3.1	42	3.2	42	3.1	49	3.6	50	3.6	51	3.6
Muscular dystrophy	63	4.7	51	3.7	48	3.5	52	3.8	54	4.0	60	4.5	65	4.8	64	4.7	70	5.1	75	5.2
Cardiac	146	10.8	146	10.6	117	8.4	102	7.5	104	7.7	72	5.4	76	5.6	78	5.7	91	6.6	50	3.5
Slipped epiphysis	24	1.7	19	1.3	28	2.0	27	2.0	30	2.2	34	2.6	26	1.9	34	2.5	33	2.4	40	2.8
Brain pathologies					33	2.4	36	2.6	41	3.0	42	3.2	27	2.0	31	2.3	34	2.5	35	2.4
Hemophilia	19	1.4	26	1.9	30	2.2	33	2.4	33	2.4	33	2.5	31	2.3	28	2.0	30	2.2	31	2.2
Legg-Perthes disease	33	2.5	26	1.9	31	2.2	27	2.0	27	2.0	29	2.2	28	2.1	27	2.0	28	2.0	30	2.1
Total Enrollment in All Special Schools	1346		1383		1390		1363		1348		1326		1358		1373		1376		1435	

* Diagnostic categories which contained less than 2.0% of the November, 1965 total enrollment in the four special schools for physically handicapped are not listed in the above table.

Patient R. K., fifteen years of age requires special shoes with inside buildup and severe heel flares to both shoes. Condition diagnosed as cerebral palsy. This child has severe valgus deformity and cannot walk or stand without aid.

Patient B. F., age thirteen. This child has spina bifida and is a crutch walker at the present time; requires special shoes and appliance therapy to prevent further marked valgus of both feet.

Patient B. F., cerebral palsy, age eighteen: this patient walks with slight aid and has severe foot problems. Left foot with severe tylomata on the fifth head plantar, left foot great toenail, fibular side, infected. It is suggested that the entire sole on the lateral side of the left foot be wedged and that nail surgery be performed for permanent correction of the problem.

Patient E. P., age ten, cerebral palsy, severe contractures to both lower extremities for the past two years. Patient has no reciprocal motion and there appears to be marked regression of total problem. No suggestions at the present time before further evaluation.

Patient G. M., age thirteen, arthrogryposis congenita. This patient had multiple surgical procedures performed during the past two years. It was suggested that a half-inch elevation be placed on right sole and heel in order to promote more equalized weight bearing.

Patient E. L., postpolio, age eleven. This patient contracted polio at two years of age with involvement of the left foot and leg. There is a leg shortage present and a talipes equinovarus deformity, plus a dropfoot of the left foot. Since this patient will have surgery performed within the next sixty days, no suggestion was made at the present time with reference to her foot problems.

Patient G. S., age ten, postpolio. This patient has a left side hemiparesis. She has a marked drop foot of the left foot with a considerable amount of fixation at the ankle. It is suggested that this patient have surgery to reduce the drop foot and stabilize the ankle.

Patient B. J., age ten, cerebral palsy. This patient also has a left hemiparesis with some drop foot. It was suggested that she be fitted with a full extension metal plate for the shoe. This plate is designed to bring correction on the foot with every step, and force the heel down on walking.

Patient D. S., age nine, postpolio. This patient has a severe valgus of the left foot with an associated drop foot. The patient wears a drop-foot brace. Knee surgery was performed one year ago. At the present time the patient could use a Roberts plate with a full extension and a 3/4" heel elevation to promote better weight bearing and walking.

These few notes indicate some of the foot problems that are constantly seen in the schools and other institutions for handicapped children. The podiatrist must take his place as a part of the team that is helping these youngsters so that they may achieve quicker and more durable rehabilitation.

3. *FOOT AND LEG PROBLEMS*
OF INFANCY AND
EARLY CHILDHOOD

(From Birth to Six Years of Age)

Heredity and Environment:

Since each parent contributes twenty three genes toward the final formation of each child, the pairing off of these genes can produce many variations in the offspring that are not directly present in either parent, but each may have been present in a former generation.

On this subject, Watson and Lowrey write as follows: "If a child is born with a deficient genetic constitution, a change in environment will not go far toward improving him. On the other hand, individuals with superior gene combinations are precisely those who may take advantage of the opportunities which environment presents to them. With increasing knowledge and improvement in technique, more and more congenital anomalies are subject to remedy or improvement. However, therapeutic measures and environmental correction cannot cure defectiveness of genes. Nature's frequent remedy for this situation is to 'neutralize' the defective genes by pairing them with normal genes from the other parent."

Environmental factors are also of the utmost importance in contributing to the health and welfare of the infant and young child. Studies have shown that geographic variations appear to be of little importance within the boundaries of the United States. The seasons of the year have a positive effect on the growth rate. Increases in weight are at a minimum in spring and early summer but reach a maximum in late summer and fall, but increases in height is greatest in the spring. The socio-economic factors are of great importance in determining the physical status of children. Children born to poor parents with poor background do not do as well physically or mentally as those born with better advantages.

To dismiss this information without making some practical application to our own specific problems would be imprudent. About ten years ago, we began to give these genetic factors some serious thought while working on the problem of talipes equinovarus. It occurred to us that if these congenital deformities were genetic in origin, then the deformity was normal for that individual—just like the color of the skin or the shape of the head. If such was the case, then it must follow that all treatments devised to create a change would be resisted. Several questions arose at this point. How long would these changes be resisted? Did the resistance to change vary in direct proportion to the degree of deformity? What can we consider normal? If a marked deformity offered resistance to change, would not a mild variation also offer resistance?

As a direct result of this work that engaged us, we were compelled to come to certain conclusions with the years that passed and now we believe these conclusions may become basic factors in our philosophy of podiatric procedure.

1. Structurally and functionally each individual has locomotive appendages that must be considered as normal for him alone. These were predetermined genetically.
2. Our standards of normal feet are determined within prescribed limits by anatomical appearance and functional adaptation.
3. Both the normal and abnormal structures will resist all efforts to bring about changes in function or structure.
4. Whenever treatment designed to bring about a change is not continued for a long enough period of time, or with too mild a degree of force—the change desired will be temporary only, and the structure will revert to its genetic tendencies.
5. Most permanent changes in structure and function can be accomplished prior to six or seven years of age. Very little or no permanent change can be produced after puberty in significant deformities. Where mild variations are concerned, some good can result with the proper treatment at any stage of life in direct proportion to the degree of that variation.

Thus, we can do much for a child with talipes equinovarus prior to six or seven years of age if that child is normal in all other respects. Should we wait before starting treatment until a later date, only surgery will give some degree of benefit. The fixation of the genetic pattern becomes too resistant to change when the structures have been allowed to function as the "normal" for that individual beyond that age.

In 1948, Thompson and his orthopedic associates reported on their findings of an examination of 600 newly born infants. By setting up very simple testing standards they came to the conclusion that fifteen per cent of these infants had pronation faults from a severe to a mild degree. Three per cent of this group had feet classified in the range of calcaneo-valgus. Excessive dorsiflexion was so pronounced in this three per cent that the fifth toe could be made to approach the fibula with ease.

It was the opinion of the Thompson group that these children (the entire fifteen per cent should receive treatment in the crib and that treatment should be continued until such time that no further symptoms remain. It was pointed out here that this fifteen per cent coincides very well with the same percentage who were found to be deficient upon presentation for examination by Army medical men during World War II.

We would like to quote from some statistics: Shands, Jr., states that out of 172,177 cases where a diagnosis was made, "acquired flatfoot" ranked fifth in frequency with 13,030 cases or eight per cent of the total and "congenital flatfoot" ranked eleventh with 2,701 cases, or one and nine tenths per cent of the total "Congenital clubfoot" ranked fourth with 14,803 cases, or nine per cent of the total. In working with infants and young children, we must be fully aware of the diseases that may attack them and the many congenital and acquired deformities that may handicap them and thereby bring them to our offices for attention. Of the many diseases that affect children, our interest should be directed primarily to those which may have an effect on the extremities.

From a broad consideration we can divide our interests into disorders of nutrition, such as obesity and malnutrition; disorders of metabolism, such as rickets and acrodynia (palms of hands and sole of feet swell—age six months to two years); disorders of the heart, such as myocarditis and subacute bacterial endocarditis; diseases of the blood, such as secondary anemia and the purpuras; diseases of the glandular system, such as hyperthyroidism, hyperpituitarism, hypopituitarism, diseases, such as influenza, epidemic encephalitis, poliomyelitis, typhoid, spinal cord, tabes dorsalis, cerebral palsy, progressive spinal muscular atrophy, multiple neuritis, post-diphtheritic paralysis, infectious diseases, such as influenza, epidemic encephalitis, poliomyelitis, typhoid fever, acute rheumatic fever, tuberculosis, and septicemia. Finally, there are the diseases of the skeletal system and the joints and bones. A more thorough knowledge and understanding of these problems is imperative to our successful treatment of infants and young children.

4. EXAMINATION OF CHILDREN

The examination of the infant or young child varies considerably from the examination of the more mature child or adult in many respects and is similar in some. Laboratory workup is similar at all ages and routine measurements can be applied with a tape measure and goniometer just as in the adult. Since the infant cannot talk and the very young child cannot be depended upon for accurate information, it is necessary to question the parents closely about the young patient.

We must always keep in mind the fact that parents bring their very young offspring to a doctor for two basic reasons: The child shows abnormal behavior tendencies or the child has feet and legs that do not appear normal to them. Whatever is wrong, the comparison is usually made with the other children in the family or with the children of friends and neighbors. For that reason, the parents will usually tell the doctor their innermost fears with reference to their child when making the appointment for the visit or with the opening remark when the doctor enters to examine the child.

It is best for us to reserve our opinions about these fears of the parents, even when it appears that they may be justified. The examination of all infants and young children, therefore, should consist of the following:

1. The routine questioning of the parents about age, weight, type of delivery, feeding and eating habits, physical adaptabilities, mental progress, illnesses, family tendencies and sleeping habits.
2. Examination of joint movements which are best conducted with the child in a supine position and should include all of the joints, including the hips. A knowledge of normal range for such age groups is very essential.

3. Examination of all muscle groups of the lower extremities to evaluate the ability of these muscles to function normally.
4. Palpitation for areas of tenderness or pain.
5. Examination of reflexes.
6. Examination of skin, temperature, color and circulation.
7. Any laboratory procedures needed.
8. X-rays of feet, knees, and pelvis, if needed.

If it is found necessary to arrange for the care and treatment of the child, we have found it best to arrange for such care on a long-time basis—preferably one year. The parents are then advised that at the end of the year, a second complete examination will be conducted and comparisons made with the original records. If the child requires further attention, the matter will be discussed in full at that time.

Office Procedure

1. The first visit to our office is very important and we arrange to give the child and parents two hours of our time.
2. At the first visit we conduct the complete examinations, take and develop X-rays, make any plaster forms that may be used for future appliances and discuss all details of the problem in full.
3. All of the work is based upon a schedule that brings the child to our office at least twelve to fifteen times during the year.
4. All mothers are given specific tasks to perform at home.
5. All children are assumed to be under the care of medical men. If they are not, we prescribe supplementary dietary care in the form of vitamins with trace minerals.

Outline of Physical Examination of Infants and Children

I.   Essential equipment.
     A. Steel tape measure—"Sterrett rule."
     B. Goniometer—6″ size.
     C. Neurological hammer.
     D. Indelible pencil.
II. Examining the pre-walking child.
     A. Have the child sit up or lie in mother's lap.
     B. Make a rapid check for normal color, temperature, and imperfections of the skin.
     C. Check each limb separately for a comparative study as follows:
        1. Length of limbs—by observation of ankle contact.

    2. Circumference of limbs at—
      (a) Waist of foot
      (b) Calf of leg
      (c) Mid thigh
    3. Measure length from anterior superior iliac spine to medial malleolus.
    4. Measure length from umbilicus to medial malleolus.

D. Check passive motion at all joints from digits to hip joints.
    1. D.F. and P.F. of hallux
    2. D.F. and P.F. of lesser toes
    3. D.F. and P.F. of foot at ankle with foot held in alignment with leg
    4. Flexion and extension of knee
    5. Flexion and extension of hip
    6. Abduction and adduction of foot at mid tarsus
    7. Abduction and adduction of foot at sub-talar joint
    8. Abduction and adduction of the limb at the hip
    9. Inward and outward rotation of the limb at the hip
   10. Flexion and extension of the limbs

E. Check active muscle activity and power by moving each part until the infant resists your efforts.

F. Check for muscle tightness
    1. Soleus and gastronemius
    2. Hamstring muscles
    3. Peroneal muscle power
    4. Anterior and posterior tibial muscle power

G. Check for normal pre-walking activities
    1. Head balance
    2. Sitting posture
    3. Creeping and crawling
    4. Reciprocal motion of legs

H. Reflex tests
    1. Test for pain sensation—pin or pinching—withdrawal reflexes
    2. Test for deep reflexes—upper motor symptoms
      (a) Babinski
      (b) Ankle clonus
      (c) Knee jerk
    3. Test for superficial plantar reflex response on heel and ball of foot

III. Examination of children 1 to 4 years of age
   A. Repeat B, C, D, F, and H of Section II.
   B. Observe child as follows:
     1. Walking
     2. Running
     3. Climbing up and down stairs
     4. Picking himself up from a sitting position—five to ten times, if possible
     5. Squatting and rising—five to ten times
   C. Observe—
     1. Width of stance
     2. Arm action
     3. Knee flexion or extension
     4. Hip waddle
     5. Foot placement
     6. Balance
     7. Head motion
     8. Squatting and rising—ten times
IV. Examination of children 4 years and over.
   A. Repeat sections B, C, D and F of Section II
   B. Repeat B and C of Section III
   C. Additional tests
     1. Have child walk on toes
     2. Have child walk on heels
     3. Have child hop on left and right foot
     4. Have child perform kick test—heel to buttocks
     5. Check for hyper-extension or hyper flexion of knees
     6. Check for genu varum
     7. Check for genu valgum
     8. Balance test—standing on one foot for 30 seconds
     9. Squatting and rising—ten times

It is very important in the examination of children to gain their confidence. Children are great imitators and it is possible at times their manner of walking will be nothing more than an aping of the way some other member of the family walks. If you can distract their attention and center their interest on something new, they will walk normally for your observation. It has also been found expedient to ask children to run because while they are running, they seem to forget about being the center of attention and the placement of their feet in contact with the ground can be judged with accuracy.

In carrying out the postural examination of children you can use the same twelve basic points of examination as were discussed in the chapter on posture. If you desire to examine them in greater detail, you can obtain further information on the child by using the tape measure on extremities and by using the goniometer to determine the degrees of motion in various joints of the body.

In conducting the examination of the foot itself in children it is well to point out to the parents that the primary interest we have in caring for the child is not in re-establishing a better shaped foot, but in giving the child a foot that will function better and maintain the superstructure above it.

Place the child on the examining stand and observe what happens to the foot and knee and the position of the pelvis when weight-bearing is shifted to the other margins of the foot. Point out to the parent how the entire bodily posture is changed when the normal weight-bearing attitude is maintained. Have the child alternate his position from normal weight-bearing on the outer margins to the ankle valgus position which is most often present in the second horizontal plane difficulties in children. The changes in the position of the ankles, the knees and the pelvis are very marked and if the hands of the operator are placed on the knees and then on the heads of the femurs, a definite rotary motion of all the structures involved can be followed. The pelvis tilts downward and forward, the femurs pull inward and the entire superstructure must compensate for this unnatural position in abnormal weight-bearing.

Because of the great involvements associated with the deficiencies of childhood, it is difficult to determine how long it will take before the maximum amount of correction can be obtained and mechanical treatment eliminated. Many factors may be associated with this time element. Since no two children can be said to have the same recuperative powers, there can be no general law governing the length of treatment. Therefore, the time element must remain an unknown factor that can only be determined by the future progress made while the child is under treatment.

We can state quite definitely that if treatment is started between three and six years of age, the results will usually be far more rapid and more satisfactory than if it is started at a later age. The average young child responds to treatment in two to five years, while in treatment that is begun after six years of age, the child will not respond completely for a period of at least five years.

The changes that take place in the structure of the body follow Wolff's law and Davis' law very closely. Because all these changes are designed to maintain the child's normal superstructure, it is very essential to have the child under observation during two-week intervals when treatment is first started and once a month during the entire period of time during which treatment is continued. Children go through such rapid stages of growth, and development that unless a close watch is maintained, harm may be done by not following the growth with changes in mechanical therapy used.

In younger children, below the twelve-to fourteen-year-age group, the most efficient type of mechanical therapy is the Whitman plate. This device, which is described elsewhere in greater detail, is primarily a lock and release action plate which does not maintain the feet in the same position at every stage of the walking step. Instead, it directs the foot into a series of normal positions as the weight of the body is propelled forward through the channels of the plate until it reaches the

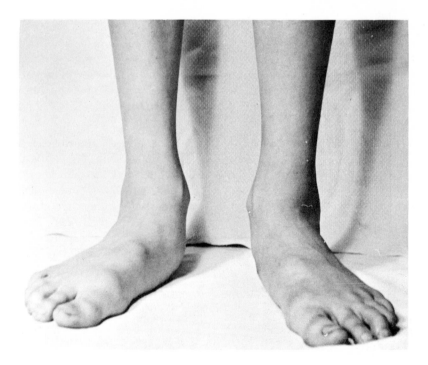

Fig. 3. Pes Planovalgus with Arthritic Manifestations in Thirteen Year Old Male.

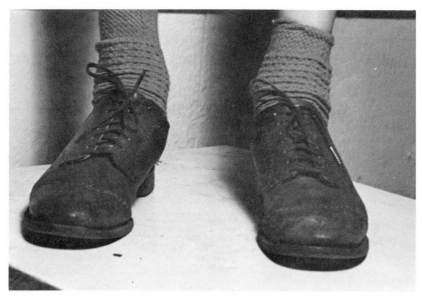

Fig. 4. Same Patient with Orthopedic Type Shoes.

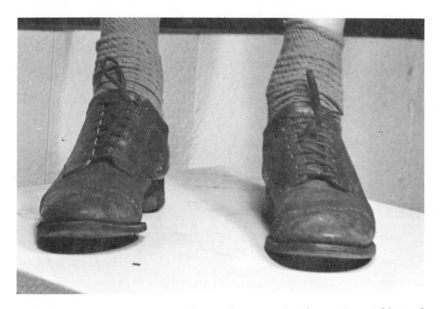

Fig. 5. Same Patient Wearing Roberts Plates Inside Shoes—Note Additional Foot and Ankle Correction.

stage and point when it becomes free from the influence of the plate itself. The action of the plate may also be compared to that of the wide meandering stream which is compelled to take the new course and flow through a narrow deep straight channel.

Another device most beneficial in adolescent children and in adults where a more static type of immobilization is desired, is the Roberts plate. This plate does not allow for the type of action and motion that we find in a Whitman. Instead it maintains the relationship between the foot and the leg without calling upon the muscles for any great amount of activity. It is easier to learn how to wear this device without discomfort and it can be worn for longer periods of time because there is not as much strain and stress as there is in the Whitman plate.

5. REFLEXES IN INFANCY

The neurological examination of infants and children is too often neglected. This is especially true with reference to the examinations for early reflexes.

One of these reflexes is known as the "Tonic neck reflex." This reflex is present in most children from birth to four months of age, but when the child is born with an upper motor neuron problem or if one of these problems should develop during early infancy, the tonic neck reflex can be activated to bring about certain motions or movements of the body when such movements cannot be initiated voluntarily. When the child or infant is in a supine position and the head is turned to one side, the arm and leg extend on the same side and the arm and leg flex on the opposite side. Thus when children are unable to move the arm or leg on one or both sides because of some brain injury, the employment of the tonic neck reflex may enable the operator to encourage subjective movement and thus begin the very act of strengthening the muscles involved.

Another reflex that is present in children from birth to four months of age is the grasp reflex. The fingers will tighten around an object that is placed in the infants grasp. If the object is not grasped it becomes apparent that there is some problem existing in the motor area of the brain.

A third reflex that is present in infants from the sixth through the twelfth month and in most instances disappears at three years of age is the "Landow's reflex." When a child is placed in a prone position, the head, trunk and legs will extend automatically. This reflex also can be used to encourage the muscles of extension that are related to the head, trunk and legs.

The "Moro embrace reflex" is present from birth to four months of age. The child is placed on a table in a supine position and either side of the table is struck with the hands of the operator at the same time. When this is done the infant's arms will be thrown out in an embrace describing an arc, intending to approach one another with a tremor. At first the fingers will extend and then clench. A similar, though markedly lesser movement, will occur in the lower extremities at the same time. Pinching the extremity of a child who is in a supine or prone position will result in a withdrawal movement of that extremity even though the child cannot carry out such a movement subjectively because of some motor damage. Stroking the foot itself with the finger or a blunt object will also bring about various reflex actions in infants and children and sometimes these actions can also be found in adults.

Stroking of the heel will usually cause plantar flexion of the foot and stroking of the sole on the forefoot will bring about dorsi-flexion of the foot. Similarly, stroking of the medial aspect of the foot will bring about adduction of the foot. Stroking the lateral aspect will bring about abduction of the foot.

Some authorities contend that the foot will indicate a predominance of movement and that when feet are held in the abducted position most of the time, any stroking initiated on the dorsum or plantar of the foot will bring about an abduction. When certain feet are in an adducted position most of the time, the same strokings may bring about an adduction. Such movements are related to dominance of abduction and adduction. While such movements are not always demonstrable as dominant reflex actions, they are of considerable interest and may lead us to a better understanding of children's foot problems.

6. MUSCLES

Muscle Testing for Infants

The palpation of muscles should play an important part in the examination of any infant or young child. When palpating a painful muscle, the child will usually flinch or cry or you may elicit a typical withdrawal reflex action. The feel of the muscle itself will give you various sensations:

1) A normal muscle is firm
2) A partially denervated muscle is ropy in consistency
3) A pseudohypertrophic muscle is rubbery
4) A hypotonic or flaccid muscle is soft
5) A polymyositic muscle feels like a stick of wood
6) A fibrositic muscle is leathery to the touch

It may require a great deal of patience to conduct a proper examination of the muscular efficiency of a child or infant, nevertheless such an examination can be conducted and, in fact, must be conducted if we are to determine what is causing a malfunction. Because infants and young children cannot carry out instructions, most of your knowledge of the muscles and their movements can be determined if you will play with the child and take note of any sudden resistance to your attempts to move the parts of the extremity.

If an infant or child has active use of the dorsiflexors and plantar flexors of the foot, moving the foot into dorsiflexion and plantar flexion rapidly or over a few moments time will give the child an opportunity to resist your movements and the very resistance will tell you a good deal about the action and power of the muscles involved. This type of activity can be applied to all muscles of the body which you may desire to test.

Exercises

Exercises are most important to the maintenance of good posture. The muscles in the trunk itself that are primarily involved in poor posture and require specific exercises are (1) the abdominals, (2) the thoracic muscles, (3) the spinal muscles, and (4) the gluteal muscles.

Abdominal retraction exercise. Place the hands under the head while you are lying in a recumbent position on a hard surface. On a count of two, retract the abdominal muscles. Hold this position for several seconds. Release on a count of two. This will eliminate the hollow in the small of the back. This exercise should be repeated six times. While remaining in this position, flex the knees on the thighs and the thighs on the abdomen slowly, then release the limbs slowly and extend them. This exercise is also performed with the hands under the head.

The third exercise in the same position is alternate straight leg raising slowly with the abdomen retracted. After the leg is raised, the leg is slowly lowered with the abdomen still retracted. This is also performed six times. An additional exercise is to have your patient lie on the face in a prone position with a pillow under the abdomen and the feet held together in a fully extended position. Again, with the hands behind the head, raise the head and shoulders away from the table. Perform this exercise six times. In order to strengthen the muscles of the back, have your patient lie over the edge of the table or bed at the pelvic line. With the hands behind the head in a clasped position, raise the body to the level of the table five or six times. This is also designed to strengthen the muscles of the back.

Test for Rectus Femoris

Tests for contracture of the rectus femoris muscle can be carried out in two positions. In the first position, the patient will lie prone on the operating table with legs fully extended. If the rectus femoris is normal, the lower limb can be flexed at the knee and the heel can approach the buttock without much difficulty. If there is a contracture, the heel will not come within thirty or forty degrees of the buttocks. In the second position, the patient can lie supine on the examining table. In this position, the leg with the suspected contracture is again flexed at the knee, attempting to touch the heel to the underside of the examining table while the opposite leg is held in a flexed position at the hip. If this maneuver cannot be accomplished we may again suspect contracture of the rectus femoris.

Abdominal Exercise

With hands on the head and knees bent, the patient can rise to a sitting position with the trunk twisted first in a side twist and then lead with the elbow to the opposite knee. This may be alternated from side to side and as a result, the lateral abdominals are called into action. Resistance is gradually applied to all these motions for strengthening of the abdominals. The trunk twists and forward bends, all given in a standing position for abdominals, are satisfactory except that in this position one is working with gravity and not against gravity, and hence one cannot develop a maximum strength of this specific muscle group without exerting the maximal pull, which would be against gravity.

Muscle Spasm

Gohrmley defines muscle spasm as a reflex protective mechanism, beyond voluntary control, by which the muscles which move the joint guard its mobility when it is injured or diseased. Phelps contends that a contraction of the hamstrings or gastrocnemius is seen resulting in flexion deformities of the knee to a mild degree. This condition is usually due to a mild cerebral birth injury or to a congenital central nervous system anomaly. The severe cases are obvious but the mild ones are often overlooked. Careful neurological examination in suspected cases will always reveal other evidences of the condition, such as hyperactive reflexes, spasticity and so forth.

Effects of Dancing

There have been reports and fears on the part of some doctors that children who perform modern dancing, toe dancing, and ballet dancing develop splayed feet or flat feet, and that if these activites are continued for a long enough period of time, these children will develop other deformities including bunions. There are no facts to substantiate this thinking. While it is true that barefoot dancing on hard floors will tend to splay the foot, in general if children are trained properly and the foot of the child is not strained by too much early activity and dancing, the strength of the foot and the structures of the foot will increase and it may actually improve the appearance of the foot. In general, the exponents of modern dancing have normal appearing feet, and seem to function very well. It must always be kept in mind that there are contributing factors to the spread of the foot, other than dancing. There may be weakness due to injury, illness, or congenital tendencies, and poor muscle tone associated with excessive weight may also cause foot problems that are not associated with dancing. We would approve of dancing for most children if the instructions are given by competent, trained personnel.

Standing tests

All of the muscles of our foot and leg are required for adequate function. As an experiment, let us consider the need of all of the muscles with reference to balance. Remove your shoes, dorsiflex your toes on both feet and then attempt to stand on your tiptoes. You will find that it is practically impossible because you are now at the stage of take-off and you cannot balance adequately with your toes dorsiflexed. In other words, it requires some fixation on the part of the digital flexors in order to maintain balance while you are on your toes. By the same token, plantarflex your toes and try to walk with your toes in the plantarflexed position; you will find that this is also almost impossible because you require the ability of extending your toes on take-off and if you cannot carry out this function, it will be quite difficult to walk properly. Try to balance yourself on one foot with the entire thrust of weight on the outer border of your foot, then try to balance yourself on one foot with the entire weight thrust on the medial aspect of the foot. You will find that this is quite difficult to accomplish because you require the three-point suspension of weight bearing for adequate balance on one foot.

Since we walk on one foot at a time, it is necessary to have this balance factor present for us to carry out our walking and weight-bearing assignment adequately. If our patients have inadequate dorsiflexors, plantarflexors, everters, or inverters, we should be able to understand quite readily why these patients are not able to function properly. We must understand the key muscle involved when these functions are inadequate. Thus, the key muscle involved when digital extension is inadequate is the extensor digitorum longus muscle. When digital flexion is inadequate, the key muscle involved is the flexor digitorum longus muscle. The key muscle in inadequate medial balance is the posterior tibial muscle, and the key muscle in lateral balance is the peroneus longus muscle. Whenever any of these muscles are pathologically involved, it is practically impossible to stabilize the foot.

Of the four muscles mentioned, we believe that an imbalance or weakness of the posterior tibial is most important, because the lateral instabilities set up by the weakness of this muscle are a real hazard to foot function and body support. The foot will assume a pronated position, and the rest of the body will be thrown out of alignment. Knee and low back pains will result from the shortening of tissue, and many other affections may follow in the superstructure.

Posterior Tibial Function

Because the posterior tibial attaches to the navicular, the calcaneus, the cuneiform bones, and the second, third, and fourth metatarsals, it provides an anchor for the entire foot and ankle. As one author has stated, it serves the same purpose that the ground floor serves for a thirty seven story building. It is primarily the posterior tibial that holds the midtarsal portion of the foot in position, and above, it balances the entire osseous structure of the body. When this muscle is weakened, it must be supported in its proper relationship to the superstructure above it and strengthened in order to prevent further weakening of the muscle and its attachments.

Strengthening Abdominal Muscles

In order to maintain the proper balance posture, there are times when it is necessary for us to strengthen the abdominal muscles. Since there are three sets of abdominal muscles—the rectus abdominus, and the external and internal oblique muscles of the abdominal wall—the exercises that are used must be devised for strengthening these three sets of muscles. This calls for specific movements which must be performed specifically in order to be most effective. The exercises we feel most efficient for this purpose has been developed by athletic trainers. With hands on the head, in a supine position, and with knees bent, the patient achieves a maximum pull on the rectus abdominus by coming to a sitting position. This is a better exercise than the traditional hooking of the feet under bars with the legs straight and the arms at the side. In this latter position, the weight of the arms eliminates some of the pull of the abdominals in the initial phase of sitting up, and the balance of the sit-up is accomplished mainly by the hip flexor muscles, so that one actually gets very little abdominal exercise.

Weak Musculature—A Case Report

Catherine D. is a nine-year-old girl who is somewhat undersized and underweight. For the past year she had been complaining of generalized foot and leg discomfort with a considerable amount of fatigue when she was required to walk more than three to four blocks at any time. Her medical history revealed that she had been under treatment for the past year for a bladder infection that had not responded well to medical care. There was no abnormality in the range of motion at the joints in the ankle, knee or hip. Digital pressure on the talonavicular articulation and on the sole of the foot did not produce any exquisite pain or tenderness. However there was pain on pressure at the triceps surae and along the anterior, posterior, and tibial muscles and the peroneal muscles. There was also pain on digital pressure in all of the muscles of the thigh.

An examination of muscle power revealed that the girl had a considerable amount of weakness in the tibial group of muscles and in the anterior group of muscles of the leg and thigh. When placed in a supine position the patient was unable to elevate her legs with the slightest amount of pressure exerted on them and subjectively without any resistance she could not elevate them more than forty-five degrees from the examining table. Neither was she able to effect abduction or adduction of her legs at the hip joints with a slight amount of resistance. This weakness in the lower extremities was not apparent in any of the upper extremities. The muscle power in her arms was adequate. Because the problem existed primarily in the lower extremities we ruled out muscle pathology of a systemic nature.

The girl was placed on leg raising exercises once each day and was asked to elevate her right leg fifteen times, the left leg fifteen times and then both legs fifteen times, and to lower them slowly after elevation. These exercises were to be performed while she was on her back, in a supine position. The mother was then instructed on aiding her in abduction and adduction exercises of the lower extremities offering a slight amount of resistance to start with. These exercises were also to be performed fifteen times, once each day. Models of her feet were made for the production of Roberts plates and radiographs were taken of her feet to determine whether there was any pathology present and to further determine the mechanical relationship of the bony structures the foot. X-rays were negative for pathology.

The patient was asked to return three weeks later for further evaluation and to have the plates fitted to the shoes and feet. At the end of three weeks there were some significant improvements in the power of all of the muscles. She was now able to elevate her legs to ninety degrees and she was further able to complete this exercise against some resistance. It was also possible for her to abduct and adduct against resistance without too much difficulty. This was accomplished despite the fact that her bladder condition had not improved significantly. The patient was able to walk to school and back again without complaints of fatigue or pain.

The appliances were fitted to her feet and shoes and she was able to wear them with a reasonable amount of comfort from the very start. As the weeks passed the patient continued to improve and after three months' time the exercises were discontinued. We expect the girl to wear the plates for the next year. At the end of the year's time a re-evaluation will be made to determine whether or not the patient should continue for a second year. With the constant improvement in the muscular functions of this girl we would consider the construction of Whitman appliances for the second year should she require any additional care after the first year's treatment. As previously stated, in order to wear Whitman plates effectively it is necessary to have good anterior and posterior tibial muscle power.

7. OUTLINE FOR DEVELOPMENT FROM BIRTH TO ADOLESCENCE

Factors That Lead to a Healthy Personality

A. A sense of belonging and security of the family.

B. Affection and love.

C. Satisfaction with the world around him.

D. The development of self-sufficiency.

E. Proper guidance towards independence.

F. Recognition of behavior patterns physically and emotionally as child passes from one stage to another with possible regressions.

G. Behavior patterns must be understood in terms of growth and mothers must know what to expect at certain ages.

H. Listening and talking to children about their problems is most important to them and to the parents.

Physical and Behavioral Characteristics of Children, Birth to Sixteen Years of Age

A. First days of life.
1. The child weighs six to nine pounds.
2. The length is nineteen to twenty-one inches.
3. The child holds the legs flexed and the hands clenched.
4. The child puckers his face and cries lustily and is able to suck.
5. The head is relatively large and the fontanels are large.
6. The eyes are slate blue.

7. The infant becomes startled and sneezes easily.
8. The jawbone may tremble.
9. Breathing is irregular and shallow.
10. The infant makes strange sounds during sleep.

B. One Month Old.
1. He has regained the weight lost at birth.
2. The infant lifts his head briefly when placed on the stomach.
3. Breathing is deeper and more regular.
4. The eyes are still slate blue.
5. The infant may move aimlessly and become cross and irritated at times.
6. The whole body of the infant moves when he is touched or lifted.

C. Four Months of Age.
1. Birth weight is doubled.
2. He has grown three to four inches.
3. The hands are clenched less often.
4. The infant follows and reaches towards objects.
5. The infant plays with his fingers and puts objects into his mouth.
6. He holds his head erect but his back still needs support.
7. He attempts to roll over.
8. He stays awake longer and at feeding time.
9. The infant sleeps all night.

D. Eight Months of Age.
1. The weight and height gains slow down.
2. Appetite increases.
3. The child rolls over, sits up and scoots along the floor.
4. The child reaches for, grasps, examines objects with his hands, eyes and mouth.
5. The child can use one hand at a time.
6. He has discovered his toes.
7. He has one or two teeth.
8. He takes two naps a day.
9. He sustains his weight when held and he bounces.

E. One to Two Years of Age.
1. Birth weight is tripled at one year and ten inches are added to growth.
2. Weight gain, growth and appetite lessen.
3. He uses thumb and forefinger in apposition to each other.
4. The eyes move in unison.
5. He takes one nap a day.

6. Sucking of fingers and mouthing all objects continue until two years of age.
7. He begins to drink from a cup and feeds himself in a fashion.
8. He controls the bowels at two years of age.
9. He begins to walk between first and second year if he has not initiated walking up to this period. Children begin to walk with their feet far apart and a broad stance. The body is tilted forward, the knees are somewhat flexed. The feet usually appear to be flat and the arms are extended away from the body in an effort to obtain better balance.

F. Two to Three Years of Age.
1. The child runs, climbs, pushes, pulls and tugs.
2. He walks upstairs one step at a time.
3. The legs often appear to be knock-kneed.
4. He feeds himself with spoon, fork and cup.
5. He develops a taste for favorite foods.
6. He has all twenty baby teeth.
7. He sleeps less and wakes easily and will remain dry all night if taken to the bathroom sometime during the night.

G. Three to Four Years of Age.
1. Gains four to six pounds and grows two to three inches.
2. He carries things without spilling.
3. He can help dress and undress himself.
4. He keeps dry during the night.
5. Right-handedness is established.
6. He alternates his feet in walking up and down stairs.

H. Four to Five Years of Age.
1. Gains weight and height as in the third year.
2. His coordination increases.
3. The child is able to master buttons and shoelaces.
4. He hops, skips and throws a ball.
5. His habits of eating, sleeping and elimination are already established.

I. Five to Six Years of Age.
1. He turns somersaults.
2. Good posture control is developed at this time.
3. The brain size is fully developed.
4. The six-year permanent molars appear.
5. He no longer depends on others for washing, dressing, eating, toilet or going to bed.
6. He begins to develop judgment.

    7. He can amuse himself alone.

    8. He accepts some household tasks.

J. Six, Seven and Eight Years of Age.
1. He grows two to three inches and gains six pounds each year.
2. He attains greater skill with his hands.
3. The knees are straight and he has outgrown his residual knock-knees or bowlegs.
4. He sleeps eleven to thirteen hours.
5. He is active, noisy and busy.
6. He enjoys group playing.
7. He develops modesty.
8. He accepts transition from home to school.

K. Nine, Ten and Eleven Years of Age.
1. He is long-legged and rangy but health should be sturdy.
2. He has a good appetite and requires ten hours of sleep.
3. He wants to acquire skills and knowledge.
4. He is a collector and hero worshipper.
5. He develops gang instincts and is influenced more by gang than by parents.
6. He wants to make his own decisions.

L. Twelve to Thirteen Years of Age.
1. At this age there is a wide difference in height and weight in both sexes.
2. Girls are beginning to go through puberty and are taller and heavier than boys.
3. Rapid muscle growth, poor posture and large appetites appear.
4. Modesty increases.
5. Interest in ideals and religion increases.
6. He wants to be like others.
7. He likes to act "fresh" to adults and the family.

M. Fourteen, Fifteen and Sixteen Years of Age.
1. This is a rapid growth period for boys.
2. Awkwardness disappears.
3. Acne is common.
4. Sleep pattern approaches that of the adult.
5. He is concerned about the future.
6. He wants to be an adult but he is still a child at the same time.
7. These children are usually all critical of their parents.

8.   POSTURE IN CHILDREN

Several decades ago, the subject of the postural development of a child received a great deal of attention. Many doctors, physical educators and hygienists were quite dogmatic about their assertion that the child should develop a form of military posture in which the head is held erect, the chest is extended, the abdomen pulled in, and all movements are executed with precision. Anyone who deviated from this posture was said to have poor posture and everywhere one heard the admonition, "Keep your head up; pull your chin in; throw your shoulders back; stick your chest out; pull your stomach in; and walk with your feet straight forward." The tendency today is to de-emphasize this military bearing in children. Most medical people today are aware of the fact that what we used to call poor posture is seldom detrimental just so long as that posture is not the result of some pathologic condition.

While it is true that we should make an effort to have a child assume good posture by which we now mean a "graceful type of erectness," we should not force all children into a particular postural attitude because we think it is right. In general, the position of posture changes with age. Most of the factors involved relate to the development of the vertebral column and to the changes in the strength of the gravity and anti-gravity muscles.

Furthermore, there is a shifting of the center of gravity of the body because the relationship of the size of the head, the trunk, and the extremities of the infant and that of the adolescent child and the mature adult are so different. For that reason the center of gravity of the child is up in the area of the thorax while the center of gravity of the adult is close to the pelvic area.

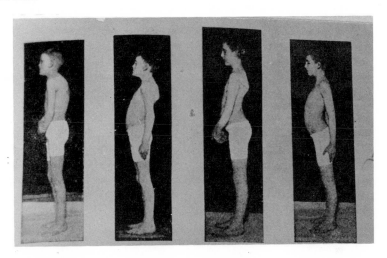

Fig. 6. Four Types of Poor Posture:
 1. Cervical and Thoracic Kyphosis.
 2, 3, and 4—Types of Lumbo-sacral Lordosis.

Because no two children develop alike or with the same rate of speed, it is impossible for all children in a certain grade or age classification to have similar postures. By the time the adolescent stage is reached, we can assume that a satisfactory posture may be said to exist if a straight line can be drawn that passes from in front of the ear, through the shoulder and the greater trochanter, to the anterior part of the longitudinal arch of the foot. With such a posture it is possible for the weight of the body to be distributed equally to the balls of both feet and from it an erect and comfortable standing position can be maintained.

In most instances, a child will adopt that posture which will make it easiest for the child to obtain proper body balance. If a child becomes fatigued in any one specific position, that child will react accordingly and change his postural attitude to overcome those forces which have brought about the fatigue. It is interesting to note that young children have no hesitancy to throw themselves to the ground and continue their activities off their feet. In many instances, this may be just a simple reaction to fatique. Only a few moments of rest is sometimes sufficient to overcome the primary factors that brought on the fatique and the child is ready to resume play once more on his feet. Social mores prevent the young adolescent and the adult from carrying out this type of practice.

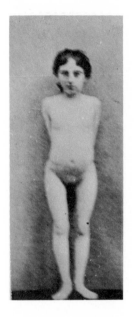 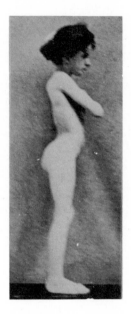 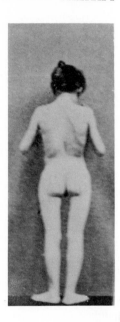

Fig. 7. Young Female with Poor Posture Resulting from Pronation and Outward Rotation of Limbs.

Certain activities keep us on our feet and keep us moving regardless of the fact that we are overly tired. When such types of fatigue set in, our postures must, of necessity, suffer. As a matter of fact, the maintenance of a military posture in the adult may be so fatiguing that it cannot be maintained for more than a few minutes at a time. Anyone who has served in the armed forces realizes the severe strain induced with such a posture when they are brought to military attention and compelled to remain in that position for a period of more than ten minutes.

Visceroptosis

Dickson states that approximately 20% of all adults develop visceroptosis. This condition is generally found in people who are known as the carniverous type. The carniverous type of individuals are most often long boned and rather thin and tall in stature. It has been the author's experience that this type individual is in most respects the adult picture of the child that showed a retarded structural physical development. While there have not been accurate statistics which would

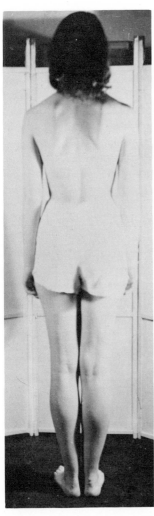

Fig. 8. Normal Posture—Young
Female—Note Foot Stance.

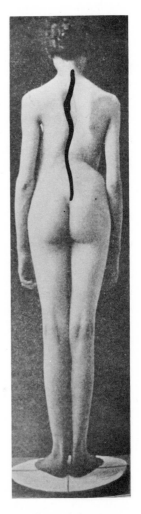

Fig. 9. Abnormal Posture—
Young Female—Scoliosis
with Low Right Shoulder
and Elevated Right Hip—
Note Marked Pronation.

definitely link these two conditions in children and in adult life, complete understanding of postural imbalance, its causes and its development
must lead us to that conclusion. Therefore, it is only logical to assume
that if we can recognize these deficiencies and care for them in early

childhood, we will be able to eliminate many of the postural difficulties which result in visceroptosis.

Even though most physicians have been advising parents that their children will outgrow foot difficulties which are apparent in early childhood, here and there we find pediatricians and general practitioners who are aware of the long range difficulties that are associated with improper weight bearing in childhood. Furthermore, those of us who are in daily contact with the parents of such children must be ready to point out these deficiencies to all who are interested.

The treatment of children who have any involvement of the lower extremity depends, of course, upon many factors and these will be discussed in succeeding chapters in this work. It might be well to point out at this stage that the physical age should be kept in mind in comparison with chronological age from early childhood well into the adult years. Many children may reach the age of puberty at eleven or twelve while others are retarded until fifteen or sixteen. These same facts pertain to the age when the young adult stops growing. There are many cases on record of adults who have continued to grow through their twenty-fifth year. Thus we observe that physical age and not chronological age is the important factor in our work.

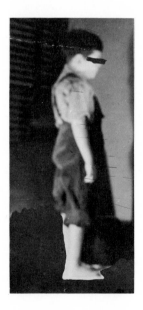

Fig. 10. Poor Posture Resulting from Rickets.

9. PREVENTION OF POSTURAL DEFORMITIES IN CHILDREN

Examinations of pre-school and school children have discovered so many instances of postural difficulties that many agencies are now studying the question of the best possible means to prevent such deformities during the early years of life. Preventative or prophylactic measures for children must be directed primarily to the parents, teachers, and others interested in the welfare of the young.

Several years ago at a White House Conference on Child Welfare, held under the direction of the Department of Public Welfare, a number of very excellent suggestions were brought forward. Many of these suggestions are incorporated in the cardinal principles for the prevention of postural deformities, which are discussed in this chapter.

First—Maintain Maximum Health

Sunshine, fresh air, water, proper discipline and regular habits are primarily essential to the health and welfare of every normal child. It is needless to point out that no child can develop normal postural habits without the proper normal systematic functioning and a child's body cannot function normally unless all of the essential elements needed by the body are furnished in adequate measure.

Second—Satisfactory Adjustment to Environment

Parents, servants, and teachers must be posture-minded and must maintain their own posture in a normal positive manner. Furthermore, high physical and intellectual standards are important in the development of best posture in a child.

Children are great mimics; they will ape their parents, their friends and occasionally strangers whom they meet on the street. If this mimicking tendency becomes exaggerated, a child may develop improper postural habits; for that reason alone children must be watched to determine how and where their postural attitudes are developing.

It is needless to stress the fact that physical and intellectual standards are important in the development of all phases of a child's life. Parents should do everything possible to encourage normal play and activity, as well as normal intellectual development. There are too many instances that can come to the mind of anyone caring for and dealing with children where abnormal physical and intellectual surroundings have led to the improper development of the child.

Third—Adequate Rest

When the infant begins to walk, there is a tendency to allow the child to remain awake for a longer period of time. The rest periods are far from adequate and a wise parent will never allow the child who is learning to walk to remain out of the crib for any prolonged period of time.

The average child from one to two years of age needs at least sixteen hours sleep and the amount of sleep thereafter should not be reduced more than one hour for each year. When the sixth year is reached, the average child should have at least twelve hours of sleep and that should be continued until puberty. For the average child, afternoon naps must be continued until the child is six years of age. If the child is suffering from any disability, either postural or physical, the afternoon nap must be continued as long as the disability remains, through the sixteenth year if necessary. In many instances even the morning hours should be broken up with a short rest period or nap. The proper sleeping position or resting position is almost as important as the rest itself. This is especially true when it is necessary to correct postural difficulties.

In the first place, pillows should never be used for infants, children and young adults. The springs and mattress must be semi-rigid and must maintain the body in a straight alignment without sagging. The position of rest must be selected with the greatest care, depending on the type of postural disability present. If the child has developed the typical kyphosis of the cervical and thoracic vertebrae, it is not wise to allow that child to rest on its back; instead it would be best to have that child lie on its stomach during the rest periods so that the back would assume a corrected lordosis position. If lordosis is present, the best position for correction would be with the child resting on its back.

While it is difficult to control the posture of infants by simple methods, there are certain types of bedclothes by means of which a child can be compelled to remain in a more or less fixed position. If children are in the habit of sleeping on their back or stomach, and if either position is not proper for the postural development of the child, constant correction to the desired position will bring results. In other words, if the child should sleep on its back in order to eliminate an abnormal amount of lordosis in the lumbar area, it will be necessary to watch the child in its sleeping habits and every time that child turns on its stomach or on its side, it should be placed on its back. If necessary, the proper sleeping bag can be obtained in which the child cannot turn over without a great deal of difficulty.

Because we spend approximately one-third of our lives in bed, adults also should not neglect this important phase of living. Constant care must be given to the proper type of bedding and the degree of postural stability that we obtain during our sleeping hours. The future will bring to light a great deal of work that has been done on postural beds and certain devices that have been incorporated in this type of bedding equipment.

Fourth—Healthful Exercises and Activities

Proper training in standing, sitting, walking and running is important in proper postural development. Exercises such as swimming, sports of all types, rhythmic dancing and gymnastics are powerful secondary factors.

Since most of our day is devoted to standing, sitting, walking and running, it is advisable for us to learn the proper postural attitudes associated with these activities. Among all of the living animals, man is the only one who does not train his young how to stand and walk properly. It would be very instructive to watch the care the lower animals take with the instruction of their young. When the baby makes his first step he is usually allowed to shift for himself on a hit or miss basis and our only concern seems to come about when he does not walk as soon as the Jones' baby next door. It is very unwise to prod the infant into standing and walking before he is ready.

As children grow a bit older, mothers notice their tendency to throw themselves on the floor or on the ground on every possible occasion. That tendency on the part of small children is quite natural. When the child becomes tired, its reaction is not different than that of the puppy dog; they will both lie down and rest for a short space before resuming

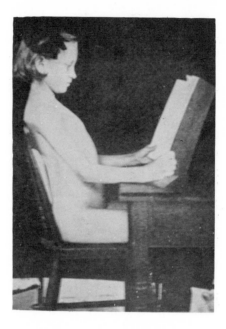

Fig. 11. Good Sitting Posture.

further activity. Therefore, the child should be encouraged to take many periods of short rest during the early stages of walking. In the same manner, a child who leaves bed after a confining illness should be treated just like an infant and should be given many periods of rest during the first few days that he is up and about.

Watch the infant the time he takes his first step. Notice the placement of the feet and the position of the knees, also the relationship of the entire body to the lower extremities. During the days when the first steps are taken the child will hold himself in a flexed and alert attitude. As time passes, and he becomes more certain of himself, this attitude should gradually disappear and the child should become more relaxed in his walking habits. During the early stages the child will fall easily and sit down very often. As time goes on these upsets will become less and less frequent. If the child shows a very slow development in gaining confidence, he should be examined carefully for some type of deformity. It is needless to say that with the beginning of the first step, the child's problems become almost enormous and the mother's responsibility grows at the same rate. Therefore, if the mother will take the

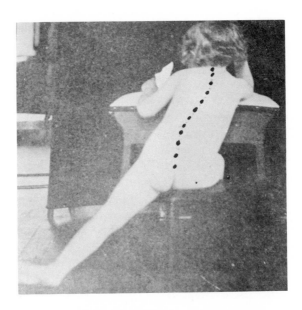

Fig. 12. Poor Sitting Posture.

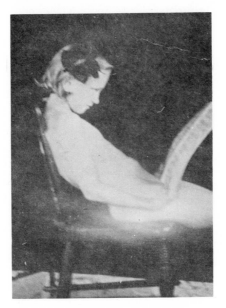

Fig. 13. Slumped Sitting Posture.

proper amount of time each day to care for the child's postural development, the task will be considerably eased.

The sitting position is just as important and sometimes more important in the infant and growing child than in the adult. While most infant high chairs are well supported for the child's back, and have an adequate footrest, there are still some on the market that do not take care of the postural needs of infants. It is wise to make a padded cushion for the child's back if the shape of the chair is not adequate. The greatest difficulty in sitting is brought about between the third and sixth year. This is the stage when the child will no longer sit in his high chair, but desires to take his place at the table with the older children and the adults. He is usually propped up on a telephone book, with his legs dangling and his back resting against thin air. After two or three minutes in this position, the child becomes very restless and parents consider him cantankerous. This situation is so common that it is impossible for all children to develop such a streak just because they have reached that stage. The only advisable cure is to obtain a junior sized posture chair for these youngsters. This chair must have a seat high enough to place the child in reach of his food, an adjustable footrest and the proper support for the back. Not only children but many parents as well will improve their tempers when such a device is obtained.

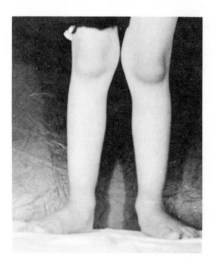 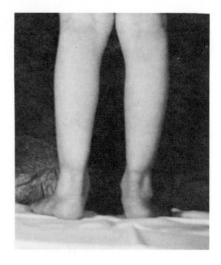

Fig. 14. Severe Pes Planovalgus Associated with Poor Posture.

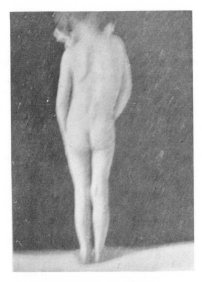

Fig. 15. "C" Curve Scoliosis.

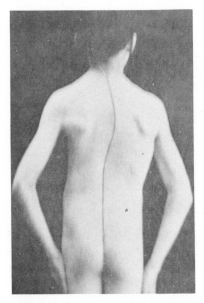

Fig. 16. "S" Curve Scoliosis.

The standing position is more difficult to endure for any period of time than either the running position or the walking position. We are all familiar with the military type of standing such as standing at attention and standing at ease with the feet spread apart. Standing at attention is most severe on the structure of the body and anyone with military experience can recall more than one occasion when strong men fell after a few minutes of standing at strict attention. The "at ease" position gives us a wider base of support and, therefore, a greater amount of stability; but even in this position a tendency remains to shift the weight from one foot to the other and brings about with it a curvature of the spine (scoliosis). The better standing position for a period of time is one in which one foot is placed forward to the side of the other so that the shift in position from weight on both feet would be to the anterior and posterior plane, thereby eliminating the tendency towards spinal curvature. This position has been adopted by our military men and is known as "parade rest." It is desirable to teach children this method of standing while watching any parades or other events for extended periods.

More work has been done on running than on any other exercise because running is one of the most ancient forms of all exercise. There is no other form of activity which offers so much stimulation to every muscle of the body and when properly supervised, running can be very beneficial in development of good posture. However, there are proper ways and improper ways of running and the child should be taught very early that he should run on his toes and not flat on his feet. The child should also be taught the value of running in a rhythmic manner, not too fast and not too slow. These little things will pay great dividends if they are attended to early enough in life.

Swimming, gymnastics, rhythmic dancing and sports should be taught by instructors who have adequate training to care for the development of these children while they are undergoing the strain necessary to become proficient in these sports. Exhaustive exercises are not of great value to children or adults and if care is not placed in the hands of the proper authorities, much harm can be done.

Fifth—Adequate Breathing

While it might sound odd that you must learn how to breathe all over again, it still is an accepted fact that most of us do not know how to breathe. Breathing should be a gentle process through the nostrils, with the air entering first the lower lungs, second the middle lungs, and third, the upper lungs. On the intake of air, lungs are the passive receptacle and the diaphram does the active work. On exhaling, the reverse is true. The diaphram becomes the receptacle and the lungs do the active work. Therefore, to breathe properly it is not wise to push out the chest, contract the diaphram and gulp in a lot of air. That seems to be the accepted Tarzan method which looks good but is of little or no value. In order to accept a maximum of fresh oxygenated air, the deepest recess of the lungs must be freed of its trapped air. Therefore, it is very important to expel all residual air before the lungs can fill up with fresh air. This requires some extra effort in exhaling and this effort must be made consciously. Improper breathing can lead to faulty nutrition, inadequate elimination and imperfect health.

The entire body depends greatly upon the oxygen intake and whenever an oxygen debt is incurred, it is a difficult matter for the body to pay off that debt. During the course of a day's activity for both children and adults, no oxygen debt should be incurred if the breathing is normal and adequate.

Sixth—Relaxation

Conscious voluntary muscle relaxation is a great asset to the maintenance of normal health, but it is very difficult to teach. If muscle relaxation can be taught in childhood, it will pay no end of dividends. Ask the child to watch a cat or a dog in the relaxed position. These animals almost play dead; their limbs and muscles are almost completely relaxed. Then teach the child to lie down and shake out each limb separately so that they also play dead. The limbs should be so relaxed that if one is lifted up, it will drop like a dead weight when it is released. The value of complete relaxation can be grasped best when we review the physiology of muscle function. Since the muscle under tension is doing work and placing a demand upon the blood content of the body, the relaxed muscle will free that much circulation and release needed blood supply to the other parts of the body. Complete relaxation, of course, will place the entire body in a state of physical rest.

Seventh—Proper Nourishment

So much has been written and said about nutrition in recent years that most patients are food and vitamin conscious to a marked degree. At the same time there must be no letup on the insistence that children take cod-liver oil or its equivalent from one month to sixteen years of age where necessary. The dosage for each child must of necessity vary with the condition under treatment. Where the child is receiving adequate medical care, these factors will be attended to.

But if the child is not under the care of a pediatrician, it is wise to have the mother give the child excessive doses, rather than stint on the amount of cod-liver oil intake.

It is now an accepted fact that postural deformities can have their inception in utero. The mother's diet in pregnancy determines to a large degree the structure of the child's bony framework. There are many instances that tend to prove this theory especially in families of more than one child where the child who is born after a healthy pregnancy develops in a normal manner during the early years while his brother or sister who is born after a pregnancy during which the mother has to forego proper diet has a difficult time during the early years of life. Postural deformity is not manifested in the newborn baby, but begins to show at the time the baby tries to sit up, crawl, stand and walk.

The inability to carry out normal activity for its age group is the first sign of deformity. It is during this stage that the mother usually becomes alarmed and seeks advice. While there are numerous tests to determine the type of deformity that may be present, it is still quite difficult to differentiate between many types of deformity at an early age. For that reason it is proper to advise constitutional care of the best type and very frequent check ups to note any further changes in the development of the deformity. If the indications of structural deformity are apparent, the child should be brought to the attention of specialists in that field at once.

Eighth—Avoid Fatigue

Fatigue, faulty posture, malnutrition and nervousness are the four primary obstacles to a healthy body in children. Each has the tendency to produce the other and all must be avoided to effect physical, mental and social harmony in the child. Fatigue must be recognized as an important factor by parents, teachers, and others in charge of the work and play of children. Steps must be taken to direct the child's attention to those activities which will eliminate and prevent excessive fatigue at all times. The fatigue factor is of such great importance to our bodily mechanism that it should be given special consideration in the examination of the child.

Ninth—Normal Foot Development

Since our work is primarily with the feet, it is almost superflous to stress normal foot development and yet it must be pointed out that while the foot is an integral part of the body as a whole, there are certain factors about its individual development that must be watched constantly. The important factors pretaining to this development are, of course, proper hygiene and podiatric care whenever necessary. If essential foot care is maintained from the earliest years of life, those habits which are formed will never be broken and the benefits will be manifold during later years.

Tenth—Sunshine and Fresh Air

Only through the medium of outdoor play can children obtain a sufficient amount of sunshine and fresh air to care for all of the body needs. The effect of sunshine and fresh air on the superficial circulation and the tone of the body tissue is very important. It is preferable to take charge of outdoor play at intervals during the day rather than encourage children to remain outdoors for long periods of time without the proper supervision. When outdoor sunshine is not available, artificial ultraviolet may be used as a substitute.

Eleventh—Psychological Factors

There are many abstract factors that have a tremendous effect upon the postural development of the normal healthy child. Some of these factors, such as faith, confidence, fear, pride, success and cheerfulness are directly related to the child's environment. The child's faith can be developed to a high degree along with confidence if supervision during the early years is carried out with the proper amount of care. Fear may be eliminated by eliminating the mention of fear in all of its forms, whether in the printed or spoken word. Children should never be frightened into carrying out a command. Pride in a child's accomplishments, in the care of the child's possessions, and in the child's entire surroundings is easily taught. Success and cheerfulness are just natural attributes to healthy normal children. All of these factors can be developed in children to a more or less high degree depending entirely upon the amount of care and the quality of care that they receive at home and at school.

Twelfth—Immediate Attention to Physical Ailments

There is no such thing as a minor ailment in a child. All physical ailments that may develop in children are major and must be treated as such by the parents and by the teachers. While it is true that children can and do show a great deal of resistance to what we consider minor ailments, the course of illness in children can run very rapidly and great dangers will be avoided if all ailments are treated immediately.

It is essential to understand the normal child before we can begin to recognize difficulties in the abnormal. It is estimated by the author that twenty per cent of all children born will have some type of inherent foot weakness, primarily associated with an underdevelopment of the ossification centers of some of the bones in the foot. If this condition is allowed to exist without proper attention, a great deal of postural harm may result. Since we are primarily interested in what will occur to the superstructure of the body from lack of proper treatment, it is important to examine the superstructure very carefully when these children come to our attention.

Therefore, the first essential requirement in the examination is to strip the child of all clothing and carry out a thorough examination of physical and postural defects. The posture of normal children changes from infancy to the adult stage. The infant who has just learned to walk will appear to be pot-bellied and sway-backed. Since the infant must consume a large amount of fluids in his daily diet, this pot-bellied and sway-back attitude is quite normal. The abdominal muscles are weak and become distended easily, carrying with them the lumbar region of the spine. As the child grows older and more solid foods are included in the diet, this typical pot-bellied appearance will gradually disappear, until it is completely lost after the puberty stage.

The small child will also have a droop-shoulder and hunched-shoulder attitude. This postural attitude is also due in part to the downward and forward pull of the abdomen on the stomach walls. Because of this great thrust, it must be pointed out to the parent that no clothing should be placed in a position where additional force will be exerted on the shoulders. Heavy clothing, involving shoulder straps or heavy overcoats for small children must be avoided entirely.

Infants and small children do not normally have kyphosis in the cervical and thoracic area. If such a condition is present, it must be considered an abnormality and the child should receive immediate attention to determine the cause.

The infant will usually walk with a hesitating, uneven gait but after the second to third year the normal child will develop a smooth walking pattern. It is not unusual for most normal children to take frequent falls, but at the same time it is abnormal for the child to fall constantly. If the child cannot control his falls during the hours of the day when he is quite wide awake he should be examined for the causes that may bring on this unstable posture.

10. ETIOLOGY OF FOOT DISEASES AND DEFORMITIES

For general purposes which may include all categories of discussion, the diseases and deformities of the foot may be broken down into approximately nine areas. These would include the diseases of bone metabolism, endocrine glands, infectious diseases, nerves, blood vessels, muscles, skin, and diseases of various etiologies not readily included in the foregoing list. While some of these diseases and deformities will be discussed in detail in this volume, let us also consider them now from the point of view of how they affect the foot; because it is almost impossible to catalogue these diseases as belonging to one single category, we will attempt to place them in the category where they are usually considered in most discussions relating to foot problems.

Under conditions relating to bone, we will consider achondroplasia, bony coalitions of the mid-tarsus of the foot, including the calcaneus, the navicular, and the talus; talipes conditions, including talipes equinovarus, talipes equino valgus, talipes calcaneus, talipes varus, talipes valgus, and talipes equinus, bony variations of the digits and the metatarsals; metatarsus varus or adductus; bifid calcaneus; osteoporosis; congenital hypopalasia of bone; congential misplacement of bone; osteitis; ostempyesis, osteogenesis imperfecta, and osteogenic sarcoma. Since our primary concern here is foot-related problems, we will not attempt to go into great detail with reference to the conditions discussed.

1. CONGENITAL ANOMALIES

Such deformities are quite common and vary from harmless extra bones in the hand or foot to very severe structural defects which inter-

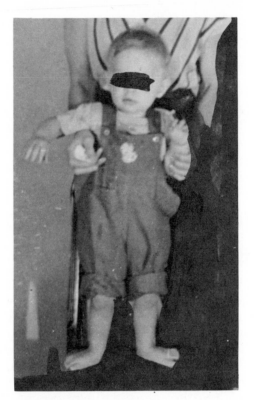

Fig. 18. Talipes Valgus.

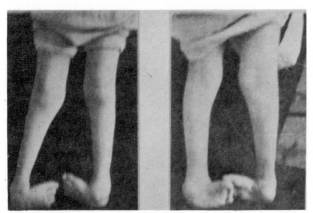

Fig. 19. Severe Talipes Equinovarus in Child—Untreated.

fere with the function of the individual through life. Most important of these to podiatrists are congenital clubfoot and dislocation of the hip.

The causes of these anomalies are as yet unknown and only in a minority of instances can the defect be traced to inherited tendency. Furthermore these anomalies are not preventable. Where hereditary tendencies are in evidence, the contemplation of marriage between such individuals should be seriously considered.

2. CONGENITAL SYPHILIS

While many prenatal syphilitics die in infancy, in most cases the infant appears healthy at birth but the symptoms crop out after several months. Such characteristic symptoms as a persistent nasal discharge, a skin rash that endures for weeks at a time, jaundice that will not disappear, or unexplainable bleeding suggests prenatal syphilis and an examination must be made for further findings. There are many instances where no symptoms whatever appear during infancy and the typical signs do not show up until middle or late childhood. While these signs are quite varied, the most important are partial blindness or deafness, Hutchinson's teeth, saber shins and chronic skin ulcers. Such children require prompt pediatric attention.

Prompt and efficient treatment of the mother if it is started by the fourth month and continued through pregnancy will usually prevent the disease from affecting the child.

3. OBSTETRICAL PARALYSIS OR BIRTH PALSY

This type of paralysis is observed immediately after birth and is the result of an injury to the locomotor centers of the brain either before, during or after delivery. Paralysis is usually most noticeable about the shoulder and arm, but may involve all extremities. The weakness of the muscles resulting from this injury makes the extremity lie motionless alongside the body. This type of paralysis is said to be an unavoidable complication of the delivery. It is claimed that the danger of its occurrence can be minimized if a competent obstetrician is in charge of the prenatal care and delivery.

4. CEREBRAL PALSY

Cerebral palsy is also a fairly common and a disabling type of paralysis which usually appears at birth.

The infant may show a number of symptoms such as inability to breathe well, cyanosis, failure to nurse, convulsions, or a definite weakness or spasticity of the muscles. Again, there may be no abnormal signs whatever at first, but the child may show a delayed ability in holding up the head, sitting and standing or walking. His movements are usually of a jerking, labored type and are executed with difficulty because the child is unable to relax his muscles normally.

The second type of cerebral palsy, known as the athetoid type, is characterized by involuntary spasmotic twisting movements which interfere with and destroy the normal fluidity of motion. Spastics are not necessarily affected mentally, although many types of cerebral palsy do affect the mind of the child.

This disease is primarily due to the absence or the destruction of certain nerve cells in the cortex of the brain. The most common cause of destruction is hemorrhage into the brain during birth or immediately following birth. The hemorrhage may come about as a result of pressure upon the infant's head during its passing through the birth canal or as the direct or indirect result of obstetrics. There are some cases that appear to be due to congenital anomalies of the central nervous system or from destruction of nerve cells by infection or toxic agents.

5.   RICKETS

Rickets is under good control in this country but is still a very disabling disease in many parts of the world. This nutritional disease of infancy usually begins from the second to the sixth month but the signs may not become apparent until the first year of life. The child finds it difficult to sit or stand and the weakened rachitic bones develop deformities because of the pull of the muscles which normal bones could withstand. Knock-knees, bowlegs, deformities of the chest and abnormal curvatures of the spine are frequently the result of rickets.

Rickets is caused by an insufficient supply of vitamin D and of sunlight. Rickets is a preventable disease and can be controlled very readily if every infant is given an adequate amount of vitamin D in the form of cod-liver oil or other preparations. A child should also receive its share of sunlight and the vitamin therapy should be continued throughout the early years of childhood.

6.   MALNUTRITION

Malnutrition may often lead to deformities associated with poor posture and by lowering the child's resistance to infection it may make the child susceptible to many diseases of the bones and joints. The undernourished child has a subnormal physical development, is below average in weight and height for his age, tires easily, is irritable, and in general is not a well child.

In most instances the causes of malnutrition are improper feeding habits, insufficient rest and sleep, inadequate or unsuitable diet and lack of sufficient outdoor exercises. Diseases of the upper respiratory organs may be contributing factors. Malnutrition may be prevented.

7. BURNS

Burns that are deep enough to destroy the layers of skin beneath the epidermis and especially the tissue situated near the joint will usually cause a deformity. The scar tissue which replaces the normal tissue does not allow for growth in the development of children and the deformity is a direct result of this inability of the tissue to stretch.

8. INFANTILE PARALYSIS

The crippling results of infantile paralysis are so well known that many deformities associated with childhood are mistaken for infantile paralysis by the general observer. However, the disease does not always leave a deformity. In fact, very many cases of infantile paralysis subside with little or no changes in the muscular tissue and nerve tissue. Where the changes affecting the foot are severe, the child is left with a flaccid paralysis and an associated drop-foot. Mild changes will produce an abduction and a limited range of motion which may go unnoticed for a period of time until development of pressure points interferes with normal function.

9. OSTEOMYELITIS

Either staphylococcus or streptococcus organisms may cause osteomyelitis which is most frequently seen in children between three and ten years of age. While the bones of the lower and upper extremities are most often affected, any of the bones of the body may be involved. In the early stages the child becomes extremely ill with a high fever, prostration, severe pain and tenderness in the area of involvement. Local swelling and redness appear after a few days. If body resistance is not sufficient to overcome the acute symptoms with the aid of treatment, pus formation must be released by operative procedure. Drainage is continued until the entire bony area is clear of necrotic debris or until such time as surgical procedure removes the affected bone tissue.

Any deep wound or infection of soft tissue may affect adjacent bone tissue and precipitate an osteomyelitis. In some instances the bacteria may come from focal infections such as occur with infected tonsils. The resulting deformity, especially in the lower extremities, is usually quite severe because of the destruction that occurs to the tissue and the inhibited growth during the period of time while the disease is making its inroads. Immediate and proper medical attention is the best preventive for this disease.

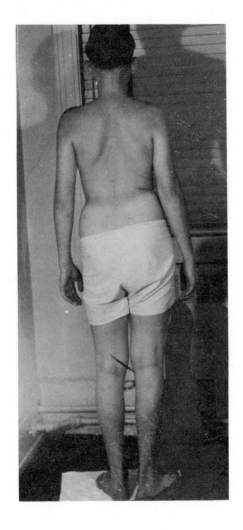

Fig. 20. Young Adult with Postural Deformity Resulting from Osteomyelitis.

10. ACUTE INFECTIONS OF JOINTS

This disease progresses very rapidly. The damage to the joint structures may result in a permanent impairment of joint function. It is due to the rapidly developing bacterial action and must be recognized immediately in order to secure the best results. Acute infections of the joints are more common in middle and late childhood than they are in infancy. The child complains of pain in the joint and the area is painful to pressure and when in motion. Swelling occurs rapidly and can easily be recognized when compared with the opposite extremity. Infections in the hip, however, are somewhat more difficult because the swelling is not readily visible. The child usually becomes acutely ill with all the signs of a bacterial infection. Again, the entrance point for the bacteria may be a cut or bruise or a focal infection of the tonsils or other organs. Prompt and thorough medical treatment is necessary when such conditions occur.

11. TUBERCULOSIS OF THE BONES AND JOINTS

This disease is still seen quite frequently in children in spite of the fact that great advances have been made in the prevention of tuberculosis. The spine is most commonly affected, and the hip or knee joints may also be involved. The disease may come on gradually over a considerable length of time and may be associated with such local symptoms as loss of weight, slight afternoon fever and poor general health. The pain which precedes the development of the deformity is usually slight and there may be an abnormal prominence on the spine in the early stages.

In tuberculosis of the hip, the first symptom may be that of limping. Special tests and X-rays are necessary before a complete diagnosis can be made. Preventive measures are the same as those used for the prevention of tuberculosis in other parts of the body. It is especially important that no child be allowed to come in contact directly or indirectly with persons who have tuberculosis of the lungs. Furthermore, any child doing poorly and who develops an afternoon fever should receive immediate attention.

12. COXA PLANA

Coxa Plana, or Legg-Perthes' disease, affects the bone of the epiphysis of the upper end of the femur (capitular epiphysis) which becomes softened and necrotic for about two years. After that period, it gradually regains its normal strength and hardness. It is very essential to protect the child's hip from weight bearing during the entire period of bone

softening or a permanent disability of the hip will result. Children between the ages of five to twelve are most susceptible and boys are more
often affected than girls. The most common early symptoms are pains
in the hip associated with a slight limp. The child's general health is
not affected. Since the cause of Coxa Plana is unknown, no preventative
measures can be offered.

13. RHEUMATOID ARTHRITIS

In general, rheumatoid arthritis is associated with enlargement of
the lymph nodes, spleen and liver. The cause of this disease is unknown,
but it is often associated with other focal infections. This type of arthritis
is a common chronic disease which often begins with acute symptoms
and may be followed by flare-ups during certain periods of its later
course. Pain, swelling and destructive changes in the joints usually are
present. If unchecked, these changes may lead to severe and crippling
deformities. The best preventive measures are associated with good general hygiene and medical care.

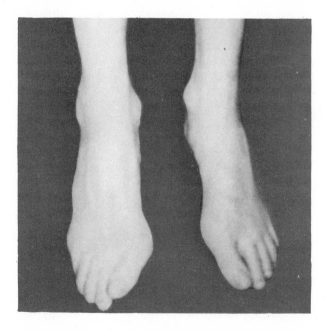

Fig. 21. Rheumatoid Arthritis—Thirteen Year Old Female—Note Enlarged
First Metatarsal Phalangeal Joints with Hallux Valgus.

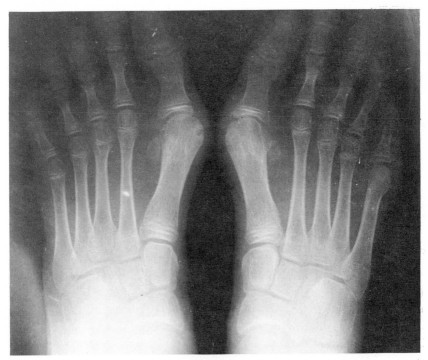

Fig. 22. Dorsal Plantar X-ray Views of Fig. 21.

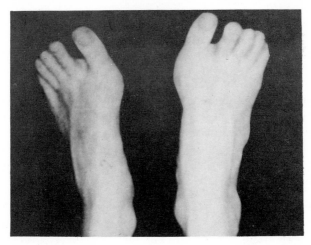

Fig. 23. Same Patient as Fig. 21—Applying Toe Spreading Exercise—After
Three Months of Treatment.

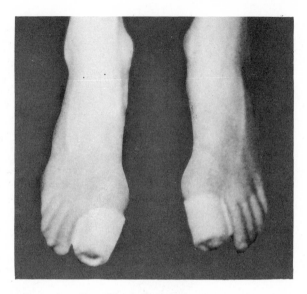

Fig. 24. Same Patient as Fig. 21—with Tubular Sponge Toe Separators Worn
    Every Day.

14. FRACTURES AND DISLOCATIONS

While incomplete fractures very seldom leave any basic deformities,
complete fractures and comminuted fractures may cause deformities
which remain through life. Joint fractures are very serious because they
always carry the risk of infection of the bone. Pathological fractures occur
frequently in bones which have been weakened by osteomyelitis, osteogenesis imperfecta or bony cysts. Such fractures may develop as a result
of trivial injuries. Complete and partial dislocations are disabling for a
short period of time but may also become serious should some bacterial
invasion occur in the joint. Children should be protected as much as
possible from any hazards that may lead to bone or joint injuries.

15. TUMORS AND CYSTS OF THE BONE

Bone tumors may be of the benign or malignant types. The benign
tumor develops gradually as a projecting nodule or mass attached to
the bone with some discomfort, but no sharp or enduring pain. The
growth of the mass is slow and surgical intervention results in a permanent cure.

Malignant bone tumors develop rapidly, cause severe and persistent pain and spread through the body. These are usually fatal despite any treatment. The etiology of bone tumors are not fully understood but it is thought in some circles that injury does play a major part. When a bone tumor appears in any child, it should receive prompt attention.

16. VERTEBRAL EPIPHYSITIS

In this disease the changes which occur in the vertebrae at puberty tend to lead to the development of an upper kyphosis deformity. Since these changes are carried out over a period of approximately three years, proper treatment during this time will often prevent a permanent deformity. The general health of the child is unaffected and the only symptoms are the gradual rounding of the back and round shoulders. Fatigue and backache may occur in a few instances. Since the cause of vertebral epiphysitis is unknown, we can only treat the symptoms when they are recognized and any adolescent child who begins to show such a deformity must receive proper attention.

11. OUTLINE OF DEFORMITIES OF THE LOWER EXTREMITY IN CHILDHOOD

I DEFORMITIES OF THE HIP

  A. Flexion deformity

    1. Characteristics:

      a. Stands with thigh bent forward at hip (flexed)

      b. Knee bent

      c. Increased lumbar curvature (lordosis)

      d. Walks on toes (equinus) of affected extremity and limps to protect involved hip

      e. There may be a twisting or rotation deformity of femur

    2. Causes:

      a. Tubercular or non-tubercular infections in or near hip joint

      b. Osteomyelitis of upper end of femur

      c. Rheumatoid arthritis of hip or sacroiliac joint

      d. Cerebral palsy—overaction of flexors of hip joint

      e. Contraction of scar tissue due to burns at hip area

      f. Fractures of hip

      g. Weakness of hip extensors due to poliomyelitis

      h. Congenital anomalies

      i. Hysteria

      j. Coxa Plana (bony head of femur becomes temporarily weakened)

   k. Acute infections of abdomen and lymph nodes in groin
      may cause temporary deformity of hip

B. Adduction deformity of hip
   1. Characteristics:
      a. Thigh cannot be swung out to the side
      b. Thigh may be crossed over normal extremity
      c. Patient stands with pelvis elevated on side of adducted hip
      d. Extremity appears shortened
      e. Lumbar spine may assume lateral curve to compensate for
         imbalance
      f. Gait is lurching and unsightly
      g. Can be associated with flexion and rotation deformity
      h. When bilateral, knees cannot be separated and scissors
         gait results
   2. Causes:
      a. Same as flexion
      b. May develop in any disabled hip to relieve pain—functional

C. Rotation deformity of hip
   1. Characteristics:
      a. Outward twisting of entire lower extremity most common
         (external rotation)
      b. Internal rotation deformity more rare
      c. Kneecap, foot and toes of affected extremity all point out-
         ward in external and inward in internal rotation
      d. Abnormal position causes an unsightly and disabling limp
   2. Causes:
      a. May be associated with flexion and adduction deformity
      b. Fractures and epiphyseal displacements cause external
         rotation deformity
      c. Dislocations (rare) cause internal rotation deformity
      d. All causes listed for flexion deformities
      e. Many minor muscle strains and inflammations

D. Abduction deformity of hip
   1. Characteristics:
      a. Thigh is bent out to the side (laterally) at junction with
         pelvis
      b. To bring affected extremity alongside the normal limb the
         pelvis must tilt downward on affected side—causing lateral
         lumbar curvature

    c. This deformity tends to cause knock-knee and flatfoot

    d. Slight adbuction causes little disability

    e. Severe abduction causes marked limp for trunk must swing far to the side to maintain balance

    f. In most instances some flexion or rotation deformity is found

II DEFORMITIES OF THE THIGH

A. Bent thigh (curvature of the thigh)—femur

  1. Characteristics:

    a. Curvature may be in any place

    b. Anterior curvature produces unsightly prominence of the front of thigh

    c. Lateral curvature produces bowleg deformity

    d. Medial curvature produces knock-knees

  2. Causes:

    a. Rickets

    b. Fractures

    c. Osteomyelitis

    d. Osteogenesis Imperfecta (brittle bones)

    e. Bone tumors or cysts

B. Shortening of the thigh

  1. Characteristics:

    a. More than one-half inch shortage causes dip in gait

    b. Knees are at same level, but pelvis is tilted and spine is curved towards opposite side to compensate

  2. Causes:

    a. Fracture

    b. Osteomyelitis

    c. Infantile paralysis

    d. Cerebral palsy

    e. Congenital dislocation of hip

    f. Congenital anomaly

    g. Legg-Perthes

C. Rotary deformity of thigh (rare)

III DEFORMITIES OF THE KNEE

A. Bent knee

  1. Characteristics:

    a. Knee is flexed

b. Patient stands with knee bent

c. Foot is in equinus

d. Pelvis is tilted downward to compensate for loss of limb length on affected side

e. Spine is curved laterally

f. Gait is awkward

g. When bilateral, patient stands with hips and knees bent— legs bent forward at ankles and spine bowed (lordosis). Gait is awkward and laborious

2. Causes:
Same as I

B. Genu varum (bowleg)

1. Characteristics:

a. Curvature may involve all levels of leg and thigh

b. Deformity most marked just below knee

c. Convexity is towards lateral aspect

d. Slight deformity is common in infancy but should become less as child grows older

2. Causes:

a. Rickets

b. Inherited tendency

c. Asymmetrical epiphyseal growth caused by injury or infection (usually unilateral)

C. Genu valgum (knock-knee)

1. Characteristics:

a. Lower extremity is curved with convexity toward inner or medial aspect

b. May be unilateral or bilateral

c. When knees are together, ankles are separated

d. When walking the leg may be twisted inward to prevent knees from striking

2. Causes:

a. Rickets

b. Inherited tendency

c. Asymmetrical epiphyseal growth caused by injury or infection

d. Infantile paralysis

e. Cerebral palsy

f. Flat or pronated feet

D. Straight knee (Ankylosis of knee in extension)
1. Characteristics:
a. Awkward in sitting position and difficulty in getting up
b. Only slight limp in walking
c. Preferable to a stiff flexed knee
2. Causes:
a. Infection in knee joint
b. Rheumatoid arthritis
c. Injuries
d. Congenital

E. Back-bent knee (hyperextension deformity)
1. Characteristics:
a. Knee region is bowed backward
b. Slap-foot gait when severe
2. Causes:
a. Slight bilateral back knee seen quite frequently in obese children—due to lax ligaments
b. Infantile paralysis
c. Fractures
d. Cerebral Palsy
e. Congenital

IV DEFORMITIES OF THE LEGS

A. Bent leg (curvature of leg)
1. Characteristics:
a. Tibia and fibula may become bent in any direction
b. Backward convexity most common
c. Bowlegs and knock-knees cause convexities lateralward
2. Causes:
a. Rickets
b. Fractures
c. Infections of bone
d. Tumors or cysts of bone
e. Congential syphilis (saber shin)

B. Short leg
1. Characteristics:
Same as short thigh, except that in standing the knee of the short leg is lower than opposite knee

12. TIBIAL TORSION AND FEMORAL TORSION

The subject of tibial torsion and femoral torsion is fraught with controversy; the 24th Edition of Dorland's Illustrated Medical Dictionary defines torsion as "the act of twisting; the condition of being twisted." Negative torsion is defined as "rotation in a counter-clockwise direction," and positive torsion as "a rotation in a clockwise direction." In the discussion of tibial torsion and femoral torsion, other terminology is also used. This is especially true with femoral torsion, where the terms anteversion and retroversion are often applied.

Dorland defines retroversion as "the tipping of an entire organ backward," and anteversion as "the tipping of an entire organ forward." If we are to use these definitions in a discussion of tibial torsion and femoral torsion we will find ourselves confused, and the confusion compounds itself when we begin to quote from the many authors who have discussed and have written about tibial torsion and femoral torsion.

The term "torsion" is actually borrowed from physics but it is not often used alone. It is used as the torsion modulus which is the ratio of a shearing stress to the corresponding shearing strain. It is also called the modulus of rigidity. From all of this we must realize that the term is not accurate and does not really describe what orthopedic men are trying to convey when they talk about tibial torsion and femoral torsion. Doctors are concerned about the relationship between the hip joint, the knee joint and the foot. At other times they are concerned about the relationship between the proximal and distal ends of the femur or the proximal and distal ends of the tibia, and in all of these relationships it is possible to have changes take place. It is our opinion, however, that most of these

75

changes are physiologically normal for the individual and where there are occasional marked variations, they are not actually pathologic but aberrations, most often due to inherited patterns or tendencies.

Here is what some authorities write about tibial torsion and femoral torsion:

In a report on eight cases of hereditary bilateral, medial, tibial torsion in four generations, Blumel and associates are among the very few investigators who describe tibial torsion as being related to the tibial bone itself. They conclude that there are two types of tibial torsion, the acquired and the congenital, and add there may be an additional type caused by rickets. In conclusion they point out genetic links, and suggest that more work be done along these lines.

Kite contends rightly that tibial torsion is usually found between the knee and the ankle, and that it is congenital or acquired. He does not confuse tibial torsion with femoral torsion. He also states that the primary complaint of the mother of the child who has medial torsion is pigeon-toeing or a bowlegged gait. When lateral torsion is involved, the complaint relates to the child being knock-kneed. Where one limb only is involved, the problem is usually acquired. He warns that cases of congenital medial torsion should not be confused with rickets because these children do not have the classic symptoms of rickets such as prominent abdomen, lumbar lordosis, and deepening of Harrison's grooves.

Knight, writing on the developmental deformities of the lower extremities, states that most newborn infants have medial tibial torsion varying from five degrees to thirty degrees, a mild bowleg deformity involving both the tibia and the femur, and knee flexion and hip flexion attitudes. He states that these attitudes should undergo spontaneous correction as long as extraneous factors do not interfere. We agree with Knight's findings, but we must disagree with his further findings that sleeping habits result in medial torsion deformities and lateral torsion deformities, such as the prone knee-chest position causing internal rotation deformities and sleeping in a frog-leg position or with extremities externally rotated causing deformities related to external rotation and valgus feet. It is our belief that children sleep in the position that they assume because such a position is most natural for them due to the restrictions of ranges of motion imposed on these children by the ligamentous attachments to the joints at birth.

Rosen and associates, in discussing the measurement of tibial and fibular torsion state that the methods of measurement are usually clinical: by inspection and palpation, tropometric, and roentgenographic. In the first two methods named, position of the patella can cause a variation in interpretation and evaluation. They prefer to use X-rays in calculating the amount of torsion present. It has long been our contention that clinical measurements have very little significance in the diagnostic procedures used to determine the presence of tibial torsion. Femoral torsion, however, can be measured with a fair degree of accuracy by clinical inspection.

A statement made by Hutter, Jr., and associates relative to tibial torsion is most interesting. In their article on tibial torsion, they write: "Tibial torsion is a phrase which has become the commonly accepted term to describe any twist or rotation of the tibia on its longitudinal axis. It has been used in connection with the rotation which frequently accompanies clubfoot, and to explain the crippling results of reductions which fail to secure proper torsional alignment in fractures of both bones of the leg. No emphasis has been placed upon the developmental changes which produce an external rotation of twenty degrees in the normal tibia or upon the functional and cosmetic handicaps which result when this rotation fails to take place. There are no reports available to show either the percentage of variations in torsional alignment in the population, or the torsional changes which may be expected during the growth period."

The lack of statistics relating to tibial torsion has long been of concern, and that is one of the reasons we must agree with those who believe that tibial torsion is not a pathological entity. It is our belief that femoral torsion is not closely related to so-called tibial torsion and should not be confused with the latter condition. Femoral torsion does exist as a pathological entity, and can be described with a fair amount of accuracy clinically and roentgenologically. Femoral torsion can also be associated with retroversion and anteversion and this may be illustrated and defined with a considerable accuracy. However, it is also our contention that the primary factors involved in so-called torsion of the femur and the associated retroversion and anteversion is closely related to rotational problems of the femur as we find them in very young infants and children. The presence of these rotational problems at birth are in most instances responsible for the development of the torsion that is found later, along with the retroversion and anteversion findings.

Crane conducted a study of seventy children who exhibited toeing-in and toeing-out problems in the presence of relatively normal feet and tibia. His only finding was the significant difference in the degree of internal and external rotation of the hips. Through X-ray studies, Crane determined that these children were found to have abnormal femoral torsion.

Aevik suggests that anteversion is greatly increased with internal rotation of the limb of more than ninety degrees, and to correct this condition he calls for a subtrochanteric rotation osteotomy. In our practice we have corrected hundreds of these problems mechanically with the use of our ambulatory derotation appliances we call "Skates." Lest some unforeseen associated problems exist with this great increase in rotation, it is our belief that this osteotomy is uncalled for and entirely unnecessary.

Aevik also contends that physiologic anteversion of the femoral head and neck axis in adults will average about twelve degrees. Pathological ranges include greater degrees of anteversion and retroversion. He believes that anteversion also depends upon the inclination of the pelvis and is greater before birth and in young children, decreasing rapidly during the first few years of life. He also states that the true angle of anteversion can be measured only on the skeleton, although a good estimate of the degree of anteversion can also be obtained roentgenologically and clinically.

Dunlap, Shands, Jr., and associates, give an interesting definition of torsion as related to the femur. "Torsion is the deformation of a body, such as a rod, which is held fast at one end and turned around on its length as an axis on the other end. The femur is comparable to a rod. The amount of twisting or torsion is determined by measuring the angle formed by the plane of the central axis of the neck with the plane of the transcondylar or fixed lower end axis. If the plane of the femoral neck axis points forward or anterior to the frontal plane, the angle of torsion is a plus angle and is referred to as anteversion, antetorsion, or anterior twist. If the plane points backward or posterior, the angle is minus and is referred to as retroversion, retrotorsion, or posterior twist.

The methods used to determine the amount of torsion present, as related in this article, include the use of a posterior-anterior roentgenogram of the pelvis, a lateral roentgenogram of the pelvis taken with the lower extremity positioned in a specially constructed apparatus with a radiopaque reference bar, and the use of a graph with a specially prepared trigonometric formula in which the calculations include the amount of flexion, abduction, rotation of the hip, the angle of inclination and the angle of the Roentgen ray on the film, plus the anterior bowing of the shaft of the femur.

Ryder and associates, in discussing the measurements of femoral anteversion, state that, "The actual technique in its present state of development is certainly open to improvement through refinement in the positioning apparatus and modifications to improve the preciseness and

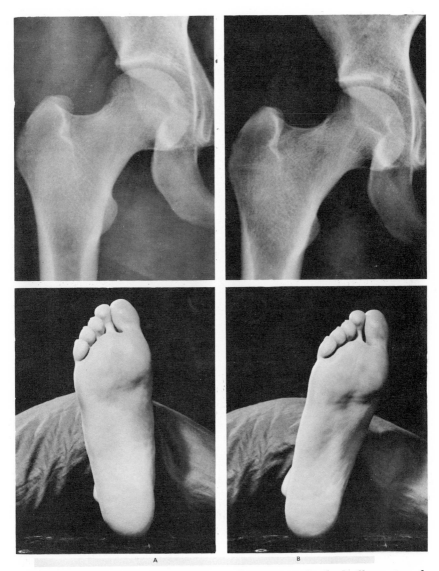

Fig. 25. Anteroposterior radiographs of the same individual, illustrating the changes in the visualized anatomy of the femur that occur when the lower extremity is rotated. The photograph beneath each radiograph illustrates the degree of rotation of the foot. A: Lower extremity in normal or anatomic position. B: Lower extremity in internally rotated 20 degrees.

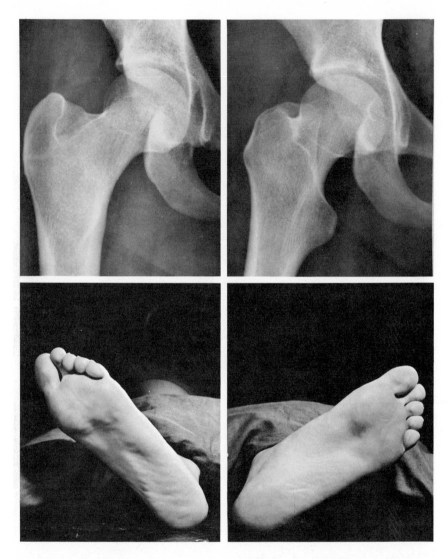

Fig. 26. C: Lower extremity in internally rotated to maximum extent. D: Lower extremity in externally rotated to maximum extent. From Medical Radiography and Photography, Published by the Radiography Markets Division, Eastman Kodak Company. Courtesy of C. F. Bridgman.

to reveal more positional errors." Their method is to use an anterior-posterior roentgenogram with the femur in neutral position, a roentgenogram of the hip with the hip and knee flexed ninety degrees and the thigh abducted thirty degrees, together with lines representing the axis of the neck and the shaft which are drawn on the developed anterior-posterior films. Further lines representing the axis of the neck and the transcondylar views are drawn on the abduction film. The two projected angles are then measured with a protractor. After they have concluded with their description, they state that, "Anteversion measurements made through the use of this technique are subject to error from two sources: inaccurate positioning of the patient when the roentgenograms are made, and inaccurate location of the axis on the roentgenograms."

Rosen, feels that the torsional axes can be determined best by angular relationship of the line drawn between two points in the proximal ends of the bones, with a line drawn between two points in the distal ends of the bones.

In taking the X-ray, the patient is in a supine position, and a standard fifteen-thirty degrees anterior projection roentgenogram is used.

These are but a few of the many suggestions made for determining the amount of torsion of the femur and its related anteversion and retroversion. A review of these techniques must lead to the ultimate conclusion that there is no uniform method which is simple and concise enough to determine the true amount of torsion or anteversion or retroversion present when an attempt is made to determine these findings roentgenographically.

Swanson makes a significant statement in his claim that external rotation deformity of the hips in infants deserves recognition and treatment to prevent a cause for later knock-knees and objectionable gait pattern in the adult. Asymmetry of the lower extremity in the adult is common, and may be attended by functional disturbances as well as cosmetic concern. In presenting a special splint for a medial tibial torsion, Barnes states that, "medial torsion of the tibia often occurs in association with other deformities such as congenital clubfoot, talipes valgus, flatfoot, and metatarsus varus. There is a paucity of information on the treatment of medial torsion of the tibia associated with flatfoot, in that they are often seen in the same patient. During treatment it is important to direct some effort to the preservation of foot balance, so that as the torsion is being corrected no other deformity will develop in the foot. The author introduces a splint that will correct medial torsion of the tibia and at the same time will hold the foot in the controlled position. The Denis-Browne splint is one which entails the possibility of producing or aggravating pre-existing pronation of the foot.

Again we must point out that we believe what the doctor considers tibial torsion is actually femoral rotation of the entire limb, and we agree that all of the foot problems mentioned above are associated with this rotational problem at times. We also agree that a Denis-Browne splint is not the ideal mechanism for correction when these conditions exist simultaneously. The primary reason for failure of the Denis-Browne in these problems is that the device is stationary and the treatment requires one that is usable in ambulation. We must take advantage of normal physiological function to bring about changes, wherever possible, and we must always remember that standing and walking are normal for the individual, and children cannot walk with these appliances.

Johanna Blumel, and associates discuss eight cases of hereditary bilateral medial tibial torsion in four generations.   These must be considered true cases of tibial   torsion,   with   illustrations   of   the roentgenograms showing true bowing of the tibias. These cases were corrected with derotation osteotomies.

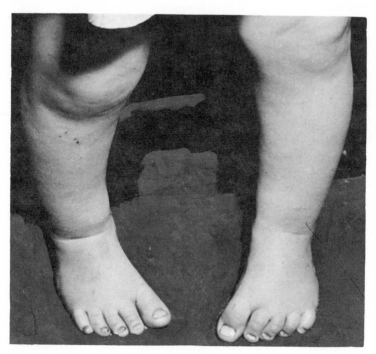

Fig. 27. Pigeon-Toeing Resulting from Rotational Problem.

13. ROTATIONAL PROBLEMS

Several years ago, Swanson, and associates published a paper on rotational deformities of the lower extremity in children and their clinical significance. In the introductory statement they expressed their concern because of the judgment required in knowing when the deformity will correct itself with growth and when it will not. They were also apprehensive about answering the questions of anxious parents of the patients. The authors expressed concern over the fact that the early chronic ligamentous strains and early osteoarthritic manifestations, seen especially in the female, might be related to the increased stresses of weight bearing seen with these deformities in infancy and childhood. It is entirely possible that their solicitude is more than realistic. If a child is allowed to continue to develop and attain adulthood with these uncorrected rotational problems, it may well be that the stresses do produce the deformities related to the arthritic manifestation.

Unlike the statements made by many pediatricians, Swanson claims that rotational deformities do not appear to improve with predictability. He states, "A child with a rotational problem will assume abnormal posture because it is easier for him to do so. The deformity, thus, becomes self-perpetuating. Physiological bowing and knock-knees in infants and small children are usually self-correcting but may become unphysiologic if a rotation deformity coexists." Swanson's paper contends that most new-born infants on clinical examination have an external rotation tendency of the hips and mild internal tibial torsion. He also contends that the hips externally rotate approximately thirty degrees more than they internally rotate but we have not found this to be true. In our examination of many hundreds of children we have found that the normal child before the age of two has a rotational factor of ninety degrees of

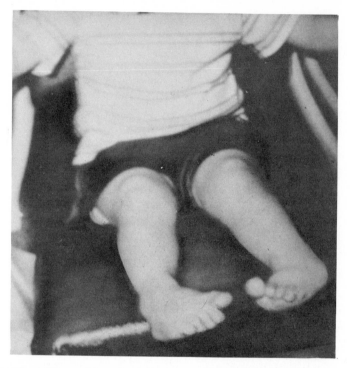

Fig. 28. Three Year Old Male with Severe Restriction of Outward Rotators.

internal rotation and ninety degree of external rotation. However, we do agree with this author that an internal rotation deformity of the hip is diagnosed when internal rotation exceeds external rotation by thirty degrees or more and conversely if external rotation exceeds internal rotation by thirty degrees or more external rotation deformity of the hip is diagnosed.

In our practice we measure this rotation in two ways. With the child in a supine position we cup the foot of the extremity to be tested in one hand and elevate the entire leg slightly off of the examining table while with the other hand we rotate the femur above the knee without applying any rotational pressure to the foot or lower limb itself. By so doing we get an actual rotation at the hip and avoid any additional rotation which may be present at the knee or ankle.

A second method is to measure outward rotation by flexing the knee and placing the foot over the opposite knee to determine outward rotation of the joint on the side to be tested. Inward rotation is measured

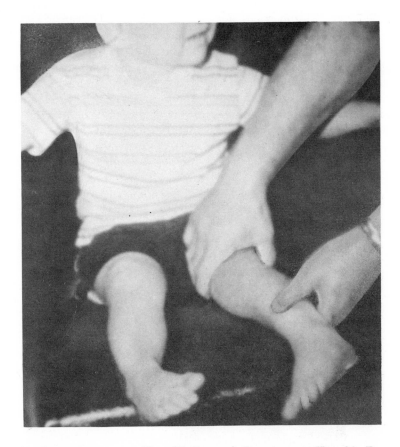

Fig. 29. Same Patient as Fig. 28—Internal Rotation at Hip—90 Degrees. Demonstrated by Rotating Thigh.

by flexing the knee and using the lower part of the leg as a pump handle to effect inward rotation, being careful at the same time to avoid any pressure at the knee itself and using the opposite hand to rotate the thigh at the hip. The illustrations below will depict both of these methods that we use.

A goniometer may be used to measure both of these movements accurately if desired.

Denis-Browne points out that the Denis-Browne bar should not be used as a treatment of choice for rotational deformities in infants and children. He contends that this bar may affect the ankles and knees before the force can be extended at the hip joint. It is our contention

that the Denis-Browne bar is not successful because it cannot be used
as an ambulatory bar, and because it must be placed in a fixed position
and does not allow for movement. While the skates that we use for
ambulation also have some residual effect upon the ankle and the knee,
we have been using this device for more than twenty-four years and
we have not found a single instance in thousands of cases where the effect
upon the ankle and knee has been of any significance and our over all
results have been consistently good.

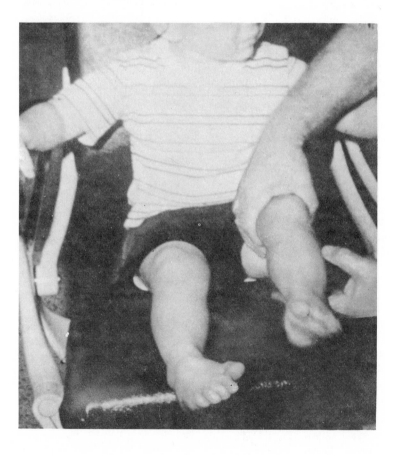

Fig. 30. Same Patient as Fig. 28—External Rotation Limited to 10 Degrees.

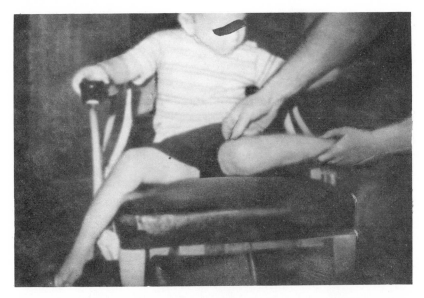

Fig. 31. Same Patient as Fig. 28—Second Method of Testing for Internal Rotation.

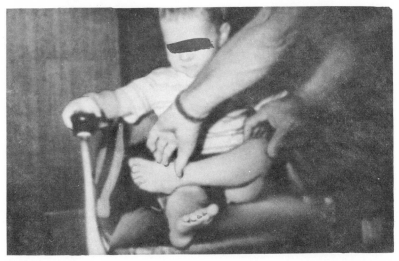

Fig. 32. Same Patient—Second Method of Testing for External Rotation.

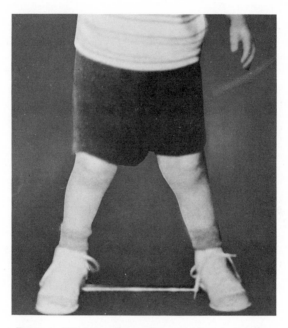

Fig. 33. Same Patient—Wearing Skates Set to Maintain Limbs in External Rotation for Correction.

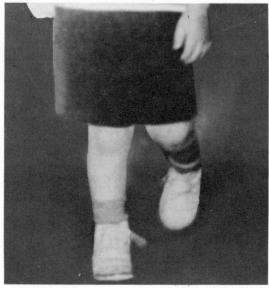

Fig. 34. Same Patient—Four Months Later after Correction Has Been Achieved.

The use of anti-rotation braces and cable twisters, such as is advocated by Swanson, have not proven to be effective over a long period of time. His suggestion that derotation osteotomies be used for children over eight years of age where the condition is severe is not justified in our experience. In fact, there have been several instances where we were asked to derotate these limbs after a derotation osteotomy had been performed and we were successful with the ambulatory skates.

In an examination of 103 student nurses at the hospital with which Swanson is associated, it was found that seventeen cases had an exaggerated rotation of more than thirty degrees and that most of these were related to an exaggeration of external rotation of the hip joint. This is a significant finding for young adults.

It was also found that of sixty children examined, only twelve had isolated foot problems; the remaining fifty-three patients had abnormalities relating to rotational problems. The most common problem was that of bilateral external rotation deformity of the hip. These accounted for twenty-one of the sixty-five cases. Seventeen of the children had internal rotation deformities of the hip. It was found that the children with unilateral deformities related to rotation were in general less severe than the bilateral cases.

The findings of Swanson and his associates in this survey are very similar to those we have found during our investigations of the past twenty years. While Swanson's findings relate to a small number of patients we must state that our findings relate to many thousands of children and adults. As a result of these findings in children we have made it a common practice to examine the rotational problems in all patients who come to our office. There have been many instances where we have been able to help these adults, especially in the correction of outward rotation problems, by means of exercises.

We must also relate that since we have been examining adult patients for these findings our results with mechanical therapy for the feet have improved considerably because there are many instances where the foot appliance itself will not have sufficient effect in compelling the patient to walk normally where the abducted gait is due primarily to a rotational problem of the hip and only secondarily to that of the foot. We have observed that there is a close association between osteoarthritic findings in the hip joints and the back and rotational problems in the adult patients. How much simpler it would have been to correct these problems when these patients were very young.

13. INTOEING AND OUT-TOEING IN INFANTS AND CHILDREN

Problems associated with intoeing and out toeing are not confined to children only although we are accustomed to place them in that category. A thorough understanding of the subject as it applies to children is invaluable in the care of adults where these conditions exist as the primary cause of foot problems.

There are four basic entities that will produce intoeing in a child:

1. Talipes equinovarus.
2. Metatarsus adductus.
3. Limitation of outward rotation in the hip joint.
4. Compensatory forefoot adduction associated with a rear foot weakness.

A child with a congenital or acquired talipes equinovarus will always walk with an intoeing gait before it is corrected because of the mechanics associated with the deformity. There are actually three deformities present. The equinus deformity produces a toe gait. The talipes deformity arises from the severe inversion of the foot where the patient appears to be walking on the lateral aspect of the ankle. The word "talipes" can be translated as "ankle foot." The varus deformity is actually an adduction involvement and results from a shortening of the tibial muscles and a weakening of the peroneal group.

Talipes Equinovarus

Talipes equinovarus is a diagnosis that can always be made without hesitation if the patient presents the picture described above and if the radiographs reveal a malpositioning of the bony structures of the foot. This is especially significant of the relative position of the talus and the calcaneus as seen in the medial-lateral views. In the normal foot both bones have typical contoured formations, with the calcaneus having

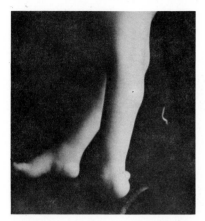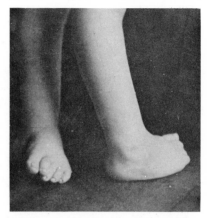

Fig. 35. Two Views of Seven Year Old Child with Talipes Equinovarus and Inward Rotational Problem.

the appearance of a Dutch wooden shoe. When the deformity is present in early childhood the calcaneus has the appearance of a rectangular block.

In the normal foot of a child the talus at its anterior inferior margain dips downward and covers the tip of the anterior superior margin of the calcaneus. In the deformed foot the talus is seen on a plane above and horizontal to the calcaneus.

Metatarsus adductus is a second factor in the broad problem of intoeing. This deformity is often called one-third of clubfoot because, in essence, that is true. It is the varus portion of the talipes equinovarus deformity, and the diagnosis can be established as follows:

1. In the foot of the unaffected child you can place your thumb at the base of the fifth metatarsal and bring the forefoot into abduction from five to ten degrees. The lateral margin of the normal foot will always be straight or somewhat concave. The foot with the varus deformity will be convex on its lateral margin and you cannot abduct the forefoot because of a primary locking or crowding at the mid-tarsus and metatarsal bases.

2. Medial-lateral X-ray views will establish a normal talus and calcaneus with a fairly normal positioning of the two bones in their relative position to each other. The dorsalplantar view, will demonstrate the typical crowding at the bases of the metatarsals together with the varus positioning of the metatarsals.

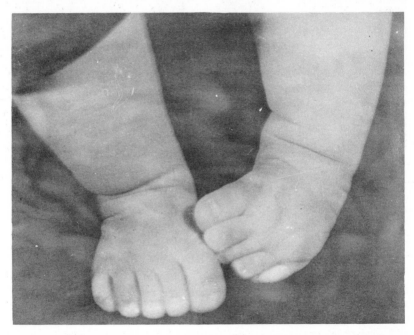

Fig. 36. Unilateral Talipes Equinovarus—Three Year Old Male.

The third basic entity that will produce intoeing we have listed as the limitation of outward rotation in the hip joint. As in the first two conditions we have described, the problem can be unilateral or bilateral. Furthermore, it can be associated with talipes equinovarus or metatarsus adductus, or it may be an entity by itself.

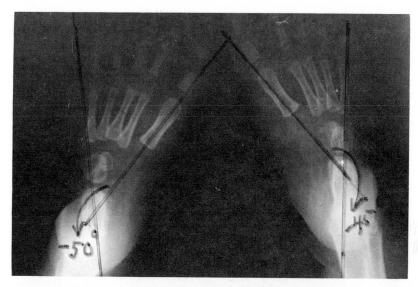

Fig. 37. Dorso Plantar X-rays of Two Year Old Male—Severe Talipes Equinovarus Prior to Treatment. Note the Lateral Positioning of the Tali and
the Crowding of the Metatarsal Bases.

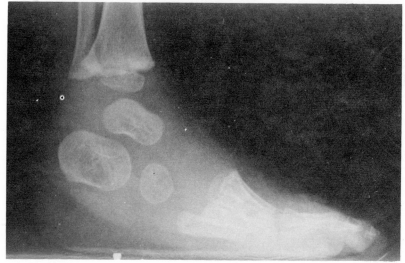

Fig. 38. Medial Lateral X-ray—Young Talipes Equinovarus Demonstrating
Block Like Formation of Talus and Calcaneus with Talus Above the
Calcaneus and in the Same Plane. Note Lateral Displacement of the
Fibula.

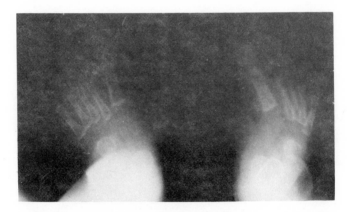

Fig. 39. Ten Month Old Male with Severe Metatarsus Adductus of Right Foot—Treated with "Skates."

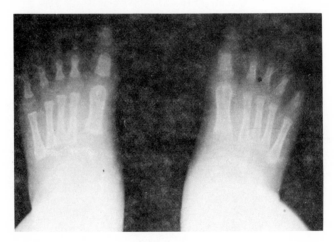

Fig. 40. Same Patient after Treatment with Skates for One Year. (X-rays from Files of Dr. J. B. Collet).

Subjectively, the child walks with an intoeing gait but none of the diagnostic factors previously described appear to be present. X-ray views are always normal. The normal range of motion for the leg as it is put through its range of motion at the hip joint is 180 degrees—ninety degrees of inward rotation and ninety degrees of outward rotation from birth to five years of age. A limitation of motion or an increase of motion within twenty degrees of that range could not be considered as abnormal but if we go beyond that we must consider some corrective measures if it interferes with normal gait.

Thus, a child who has a range of sixty degrees of outward rotation and one hundred twenty degrees of inward rotation will walk with an intoeing gait because the placement of the foot depends primarily upon the pendulum-like swing of the entire limb. It is our opinion that the primary pathology lies in the ligaments of the hip joints, specifically in the pubocapsular ligament and the ischiocapsular ligament. A shortened pubocapsular ligament at birth will induce an intoeing gait because motion in the range of outward rotation will be limited.

The reverse is also true with reference to the relationship between the ischiocapsular ligament and out-toeing gait, as we shall see later. It may also be sufficient here to state that special shoes, built-up shoes and foot appliances as such are of little or no value in correcting this condition.

Compensatory Intoeing

The fourth basic entity that will produce intoeing is listed as a compensatory forefoot adduction associated with a rearfoot weakness. This entity is most important and it is the least understood. Knowledge of this condition will clear away a great deal of confusion that has existed in the past about the basic intoeing problems commonly seen.

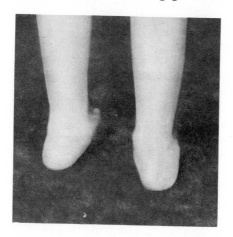

Fig. 41. Rear View of Child with Compensatory Pigeontoeing.

Objectively, these children will present a marked Helbing's sign associated with rearfoot weakness and a forefoot that adducts when the child is walking. There is no crowding at the metatarsal bases and all X-ray findings are fairly normal, or they may demonstrate a retardation in bony development. The question may well be asked, "Why do these children pigeon-toe while all other children with rear foot problems adduct the forefoot?"

It is our opinion that these children have excellent anterior and posterior tibial muscular action and they toe in reflexly or instinctively to overcome the rear foot weakness.

It may be that weight bearing with the rear foot in valgus produces a pain reflex that activates the tibials similar to the action obtained by applying digital pressure at the talonavicular articulation. These children are fore-shortening the longitudinal arch and thus bringing about the same foot attitude that we strive for when we strap the foot or pad the shoe or use a Whitman plate to correct a "weak foot" problem.

It is obvious, therefore, that we must aid these children in their valiant efforts to accommodate for this condition and do all that we can to help them walk with an intoeing gait until such a time when the structures are strong enough to carry the body weight without undue strain on the rear foot. That may take a number of years to effect, but the parents must be instructed as to the apparently contradictory gait problem involved.

Out-toeing Problems

Out-toeing problems have been divided into four basic categories.
1. Talipes equinovalgus
2. Talipes calcaneovalgus
3. Limitation of inward rotation in the hip joint.
4. Calcaneovalgus

A congenital talipes equinovalgus gait or the acquired deformity of the same type is always an out-toeing gait. This deformity can be best described by stating that it is the opposite of talipes equinovarus. The child walks with the foot in marked valgus and abducted, but on the toes. The peroneal muscles are shortened and the tibial muscles are weak and inadequate, allowing the foot to be pulled into a valgus and abducted position.

X-rays of this condition will reveal structural changes in the tarsal bones as well as a malpositioning of the bones of the foot. The primary variation from the X-ray of a talipes equinovarus foot will be the talocalcaneal relationship. In this deformity the talus will appear to be in an almost vertical line to the calcaneus, almost anterior and at right angles to it.

Talipes Calcaneovalgus

Talipes calcaneovalgus, the second of the four basic entities that will produce outtoeing, is very similar to that of talipes equinovalgus except for the fact that the child walks with the toes high off the floor and only the heel touches. In this condition the extensors are shortened and the flexors are weak and inadequate.

Both of the conditions described above are uncommon and in recent years appear to be lessening in frequency.

Rotational Factors

The third basic entity that produces outtoeing the limitation of inward rotation in the hip joint, is observed with great frequency and is a finding that can produce considerable foot problems if it is not corrected. These problems are usually associated with structural deficiencies that develop during the early formative stages because of improper weight bearing attitude.

This condition may also be associated with talipes equinovalgus or talipes calcaneovalgus. Nevertheless, it must be recognized as a separate entity and treated accordingly.

It is our opinion that a congenital shortening of the ischiocapsular ligament is the original and primary etiological factor. This shortening precludes full rotation of the limb in the normal range of internal rotation. The author has seen many patients less than one year of age who have 180 degrees of outward rotation and no inward rotation whatever. When these children begin to stand and walk they hold their feet and legs at a ninety degree position with the plane of foreward progression.

Most of the problems in this category are bilateral, only occasionally unilateral. Many problems of limitation of rotation at the hip are associated with brain injuries, such as cerebral palsy.

Analysis of Rotational Factors

It is our belief that locomotion is initiated from the hip joint and the position that the foot takes in its relationship to the walking surface depends almost entirely upon the relationship of the limb to the hip joint. Thus, if the limb is maintained in a position of outward rotation,

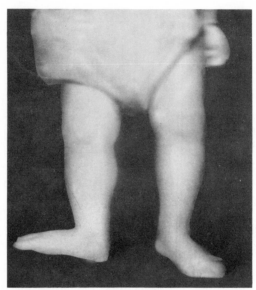

Fig. 42. Talipes   Valgus—Severe—Two   Year
Old Male.

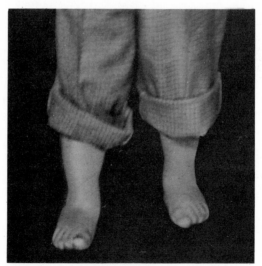

Fig. 43. Same Patient after Treatment with
"Skates" for Two Years.

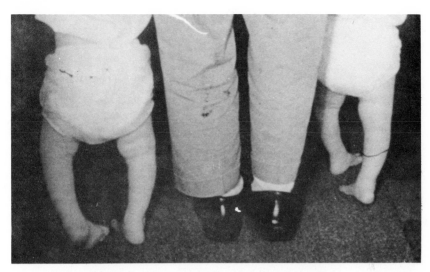

Fig. 44. Two Year Old Twin Females with Marked Intoeing, Genu Varum and Scissor's Gaits. Originally Diagnosed as Tibial Torsion and Knee Involvement.

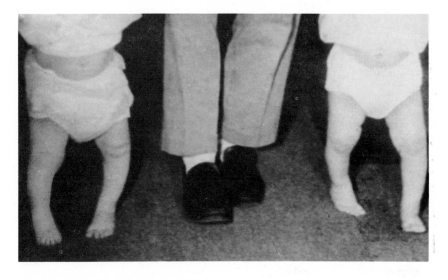

Fig. 45. Same Twins—Anterior View.

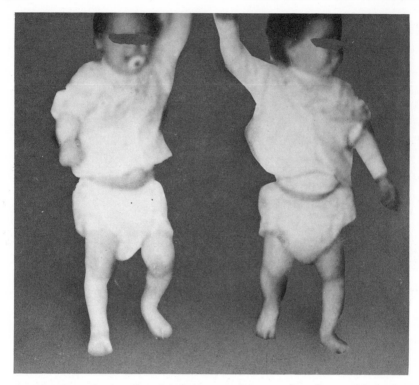

Fig. 46. Same Twins after Condition was Diagnosed as Severe Limitation of
        Outward Rotation and Infants Were Treated with Skates, after Six
        Months. Skates Were Worn Full Time All Day Long with No Night
        Wear.

the foot itself will most often be outwardly rotated in its relationship to
the leg. Conversely, if the limb is maintained in a position of inward
rotation, the foot will be rotated inward.

    This tendency toward inward rotation, outward rotation, or what
may be considered the normal range, is present at birth and if nothing
interferes with this position, it is maintained more or less as the child
grows older.

It can be estabished that the normal range of motion of the limb at the hip joint in total inward and outward rotation is approximately 180 degrees, of which ninety degrees are in the range of inward and ninety degrees in the range of outward rotation. Since we must allow for variations that could fall within normal limits we could also allow a ten degree variation either way without considering it as being beyond the normal range. Thus, if the range of inward rotation of a limb was 100 degrees and that of outward rotation was eighty degrees we would consider that to be within normal limits, but if the range of inward rotation was 130 degrees and the range of outward rotation was fifty degrees, we would consider that abnormal and not conducive to normal function.

These variations are found not only in children but also in adults of all ages, and the degree of variations range almost through the entire scale of 360 degrees. In recent years it has been less than conceivable for us to assume that we can overcome the placement of the foot in abduction or adduction without first considering the basic hip problem and determining what can be done with it.

To return once more to the condition as found in children, it becomes fairly obvious that if the child is allowed to persist in this abnormal placement of the limbs, Newton's third law of motion must become operative and foot deformity must result. Since this, in our opinion, is a most important finding, let us analyze the anatomical factors in connection with the hip joint which contribute to this thesis.

Acetabulum

In this analysis, we will review the development of the acetabulum, the development of the head of the femur, the structures surrounding the femur and the ligaments and muscles that are so basic in maintaining the rotational position of the femur, which in turn controls the position of the limb itself.

The proximal end of the femur ossifies from three centers. The head of the femur begins to ossify during the second half of the first year after birth and becomes completely joined to the neck during the nineteenth year. The greater trochanter appears about the fourth year and unites with the shaft at about the eighteenth year. The lesser trochanter appears at the fourth year and is united the seventeenth year. Both trochanters are considered part of the joint area because they are contained within the capsule of the hip joint.

The acetabulum itself is ossified from three primary centers. These centers converge at thirteen or fourteen but do not unite until the twentieth to twenty-fourth year.

The femoral head is usually rounded to conform to the acetabulum. If the acetabulum is deep the head may become elongated and pointed and the fovea may be absent. In congenital dislocation the head may be completely eroded or mushroom-shaped. There may be grooves in the head resulting from pressure by a fold in the articular cartilage.

In congenital dislocation of the hip the lesser trochanter may also be absent or flattened out.

A decrease in the angle of inclination between the head and neck and the shaft of the femur (coxa vara) may be due to trauma, slipped epiphysis, or disease. An increase (coxa valga) may be due to disuse paralysis of the lower extremity where there is little or no weight bearing. This angle is considerably greater in all children than in the adult and decreases with age as weight bearing increases.

The acetabulum may be narrow, wide, eliptical, large or small. It may also vary in depth and may be so shallow that the head is barely supported or so deep that motion is limited. The acetabular floor may protrude into the pelvic cavity. If the superior portion of the rim is not well developed, or if it is flattened, dislocation of the head may result. The displaced femoral head may create a false acetabulum on the outside of the ilium. In cases of dislocation facets may develop on the posterior acetabular rim from pressure and friction against the lesser trochanter.

Hip Ligaments

The ligaments of the hip joint play a most important part in our thesis. Primarily, these ligaments are the pubofemoral capsular ligament, the ischiofemoral capsular ligament and the iliofemoral ligament, sometimes known as the "Y" ligament of Bigelow. The lesser ligaments within the acetabulum itself are also of some importance. These include the ligamentum teres, the transverse ligament and the labrum glenoidale or cotyloid ligament.

The pubofemoral capsular ligament runs from the ramus of the pubis to the pubic part of the acetabular margin and in this position it limits outward rotation of the femur. The ischiofemoral capsular ligament runs from the ramus of the ischium to the ischial part of the acetabular margin and lies at the posterior aspect of the joint. From this position its primary purpose is to limit inward rotation of the femur.

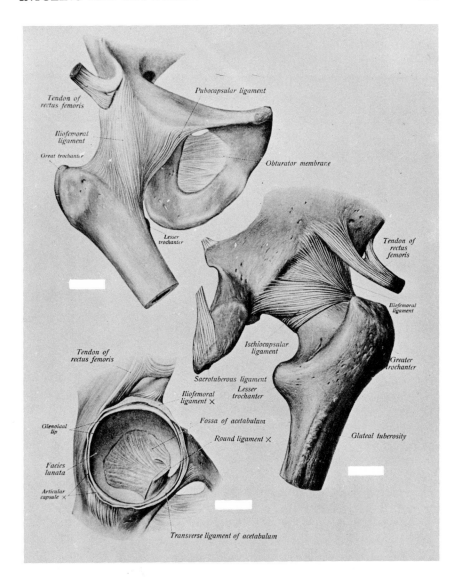

Fig. 47. (Hip Joint).

The iliofemoral or "Y" ligament of Bigelow forms an inverted Y and attaches above to the anterior inferior iliac spine and to the acetabular margin for two and one half inches behind it. It is coextensive with the rectus femoris, and, with the vastus medialis, it creates the trochanteric line. The upper limb of the iliofemoral ligament also aids in the limitation of lateral rotation.

The ligamentum teres is a strong, somewhat flattened band of fibrous tissue, attached by one end to the superior half of the depression on the head of the femur and by its medial end to the lower edge of the articular surface of the transverse ligament. This ligament varies greatly in its strength and development in different subjects and in certain cases it is absent. The ligamentum teres is usually tense when the femur is rotated laterally, and by so doing it also aids in the restriction of lateral rotation.

The transverse ligament bridges the acetabular notch and consists of strong transverse fibres which are attached to both of its margins, but more extensively to the postero-inferior margin.

The labrum glenoidal or cotyloid ligament consists of a strong ring of fibrocartilaginous tissue attached to the entire rim of the cup. This ligament grasps the head of the femur which it encircles and is firmly implanted on the rim of the acetabulum and the transverse ligament.

An articular capsule completely invests the joint cavity. Its fibrous stratum is of great strength although it is not of equal thickness throughout, being considerably thicker on the supra-anterior aspect than at any other part.

The primary muscles that aid in the inward rotation of the femur on weight bearing are the iliopsoas, the pectineus and the adductor longus. The primary outward rotators of the femur are the gluteus maximus and the short muscles of the thigh which include the piriformis, obturator internus, gemelli, obturator externus and the quadratus femoris. It will be observed at once that the outward rotators are far more powerful than the inward rotators, but they are balanced in some degree by the ligaments which limit outward rotation.

A rapid review of the anatomical structure of the hip joint shows that it is constructed not so much to allow great freedom of movement such as the shoulder joint, but for stability, which is so essential in the maintenance of the erect attitude. It is also apparent that the range of motion that is present is checked very well by balances and counterbalances. However, it is this balance phase of the hip joint that gives us the primary cause for concern because whenever it is disturbed by individual variations which are present at birth, a basic balance problem in the feet will result.

Fortunately, this abnormality which can exist in the normal with a rotational problem, as is often the case, can be corrected with skate therapy with a considerable degree of effectiveness and with lasting results.

Where the problems are less severe, the use of passive exercises, massage, manipulation and simple bar type night splints are all very effective if they are started at an early age. If standing and walking has already been initiated, it may be well to stress some form of mechanical foot therapy such as foot plates or shoe corrections for milder conditions.

Shoes by themselves are not therapeutic for hip problems and those shoes which have some so-called therapuetic factors built into them must be used with discretion. In fact, most of them have only such devices that do not harm but also do very little good. In the main, these children need specific therapy and shoes are non-specific. However, it is important that all children's shoes be fitted properly for length and width.

Whenever it is necessary to treat the problem of calcaneovalgus in children past five or six years of age, all modalities can be called into use to the fullest measure. Often, strapping, physical therapy and specific dancing techniques are of direct value.

14. *THE USE OF THE BRACHMAN SKATES IN THE TREATMENT OF FOOT PROBLEMS IN EARLY CHILDHOOD*

In 1947 our paper, "A New and Original Development in the Treatment of Talipes Equinovarus," was presented for publication in the N. A. C. Journal and it was published in July 1948. This paper was confined to the use of these ambulatory skates in the care and treatment of forty-six cases of talipes equinovarus by myself and ten colleagues. Thirty-six of these cases were treated by the author personally. Five children in this group of thirty-six were referred for treatment by Robert T. McElvenny, an orthopedic surgeon, and were treated with his cooperative assistance.

For more than a year prior to the writing of this paper we had started to use the skates in conditions other than true talipes. These early trials were so successful that from 1948 to 1954 the skates were used in more than 300 cases of calcaneovalgus, metatarsus adductus, rotation abnormalities of the lower extremities involving the hip joints, and cerebral palsy.

While each of the involvements listed has individual characteristics that have very little in common with each other, they all have one factor in common, and that is each of them interferes radically with the ability of the child to stand and walk in a normal manner. It is that common factor that the skates are able to correct for two basic reasons.

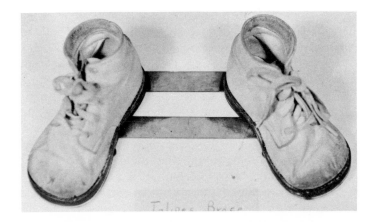

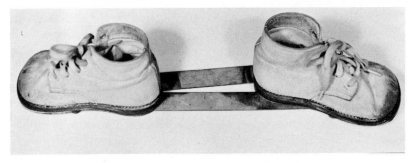

Fig. 48. Two Views of Double Bar "Skates" Used for Many Years. Every
Pair was Custom Made to Order and Use Was Therefore Limited.

1. The skates provide a broad base of support that have almost
   ten times the square inch area of the average single shoe sole
   of a young child. That alone enables some of these children to
   stand and walk who have not been able to do so before.

2. The skates provide for movements approaching the normal under physiological conditions that simulate the normal gait; in
   other words, the treatment is ambulatory and fits in perfectly with
   the entire basis for the existence of podiatry as a profession.

The illustrations Fig. 49, depict the author's talipes brace which, if applied and used according to directions, will overcome both primary clubfoot deformity and eliminate most of the malfunction which is usually associated with other treatments. This device should be applied at three months of age to the average case of talipes. During the first three months the condition should be treated by strapping and manipulation. In severe problems the device must be worn day and night until the child is approximately two years of age and walking must not be attempted without the device before that time. An accurate check and X-ray records should be kept during this period of treatment. If the child has a retarded bony development, such as may occur even in normal feet and does occur in most clubfoot victims, walking should be delayed beyond the second year.

The child can be encouraged to crawl, stand, and even walk as long as the device is used. The angle of correction on the device should be adjusted from time to time as may be deemed necessary.

It will be observed that the author's concept relating the relationship of the rotary muscles of the thigh to the clubfoot is further strengthened by the fact that this special device has a primary effect on these muscles. If the average case of talipes equinovarus is observed closely during the treatment period of the first three months, it will be noticed that most of the deformity relating to the foot itself can be eliminated by strapping, massaging and manipulation. However, the adduction cannot be eliminated in this manner and this is true only because of the involvement of the rotary muscles and ligaments of the thigh prevent the treatment from having the desired effect. That is also the reason for the return of the complete deformity when treatment is stopped after an apparent correction.

The persistence in the adducted position makes it simple for the foot to again assume an inverted and equinus position also. After the child begins to walk, the talipes device should be continued as a rest splint during the afternoon rest period and as a night splint. The length of time for this continuous use is, of course, dependent upon the results obtained and it may be necessary to use it, in some instances, to the twelfth year. The talipes brace is simple to apply and should be changed as often as it is necessary to change the shoe size. From a treatment standpoint, from the results obtained, and also from an economic consideration, it will be found to be the most logical answer for clubfoot therapy.

The talipes brace can be applied for the varus or valgus condition. The child is allowed full motion in the over-corrected position but the feet are not allowed to come back into the abnormal position. There is also the walking stroke up to eight inches so that the child can shuffle and get all primary foot and leg motions except lifting the feet off the floor. The device holds the feet and limb in an over-corrected position while the child is carrying out most normal weight-bearing and walking functions.

To the present time, all types of clubfoot conditions, ranging from children three months of age to children eight years of age, have shown excellent results with its use. There have been no failures and even in those children who had received inadequate treatment in infancy, the brace worked very well. Of particular interest is the manner in which this brace overcomes the calcaneal varus and enables the heel to come down into normal contact with the ground. The revised brace is simple to attach to shoes and easily adjusted by the doctor.

Denis-Browne Bar

Milton H. Krantz states that the Denis-Browne bar is an efficient instrument for the treatment of limb rotations, and that the device should be carefully prepared and managed to fit the needs of each case in which it is used. Krantz's discussion on the treatment of gait rotations with the Denis-Browne bar is of considerable interest to those who have used this device for the treatment of children's foot problems. The Denis-Browne bar can be an effective instrument in the hands of any doctor who has made a thorough study of its possibilities and who retains close and intimate contact with the parents of the children he is treating. However, there are numerous instances where such bars are applied by shoe stores where the patients have been sent by the pediatricians or other doctors for such application, and the therapy then falls in the hands of the shoe men.

It is most difficult to compete with such misapplication of what should have been professional service. Furthermore, as we have pointed out previously, the Denis-Browne bar fixes the feet and legs in a predetermined position, and that position remains until it is changed by the parents, the shoe men or the doctor. It is easy to change this position by the simple manipulation of the butterfly nut, and, in many instances, the value of this device has been utterly defeated because of this inept doctoring.

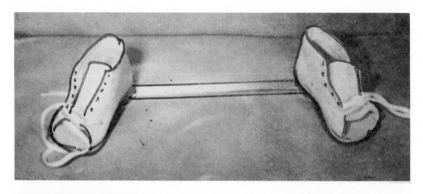

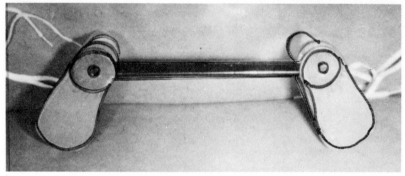

Fig. 49. Single Bar "Skates" Which Can be Applied by Doctor or Assistant and Corrections Made Within Minutes.

Calcaneovalgus

The term calcaneovalgus is used to cover what most of us have been calling severe infantile or juvenile weak foot or pronation syndrome. If, when examining an infant or a young child, you find that you can dorsiflex the foot with such ease that the fifth toe touches the shaft of the fibula and plantar flexion is limited, you are dealing with a positive calcaneovalgus. Two per cent of all children have this finding at birth to such a degree that they require drastic treatment as early as possible, preferably before six years of age. Unless these involvements

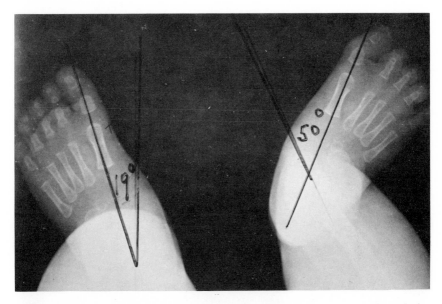

Fig. 50. Xrays of Unilateral Calcaneovalgus. Note Correction Effected for Right Foot with Use of "Skates" for Six Months.

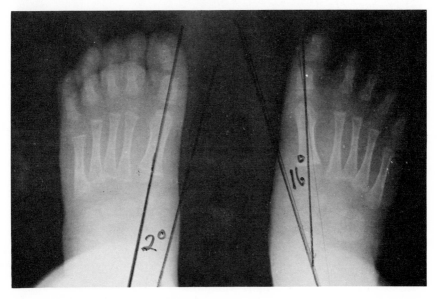

Fig. 51. Same X-rays after Correction.

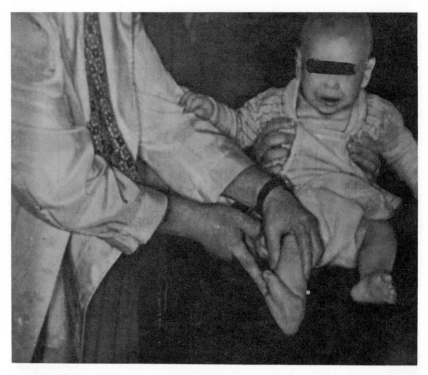

Fig. 52. Testing for Calcaneovalgus in Seven Months Old Child. Note that
    Dorsum of Foot Touches the Fibula with Ease. Plantar Flexion is
    Limited.

are treated early, the foot condition is retained for life regardless of
the type of foot care applied at a later date. Fifteen per cent of all
children have this condition to some degree at birth but these children can usually be aided by other therapy. Even these children should
also be cared for as early as possible.

In many instances this problem of calcaneovalgus may be further
complicated with a rotation abnormality at the hip involving an exaggeration of outward rotation and a limitation of inward rotation. In most
of these calcaneovalgus problems we can obtain full correction with the

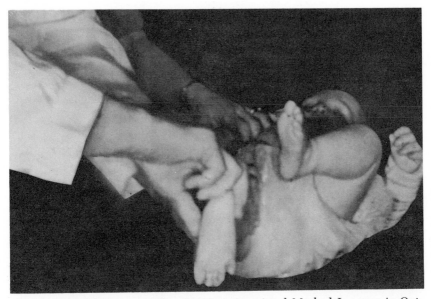

Fig. 53. Same Patient as in Fig. 52. Note Associated Marked Increase in Outward Rotation—180°.

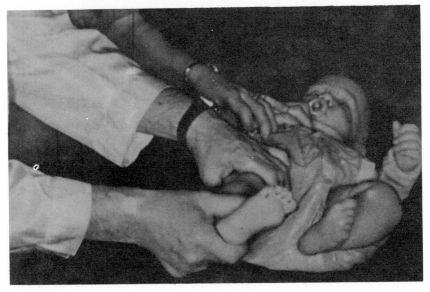

Fig. 54. Same Patient—Note Marked Limitation of Inward Rotation—45°.

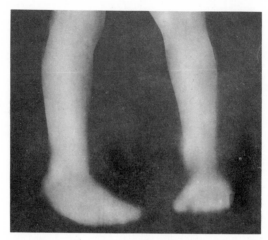

Fig. 55.   Metatarsus Adductus—Five Year Old
Male.

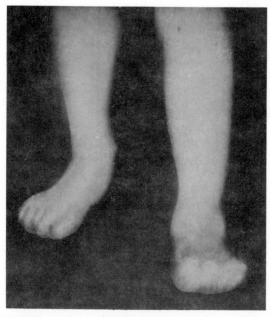

Fig. 56.   Same Patient Four Months Later—
Treatment with Skates Only.

skates in a period of three months. After the skates have been removed, no further treatment is needed in most instances. Our series of cases now include a number of children we have followed for twenty years after the original treatment. Some of these we recorded on moving picture films showing them as the years go by. As yet we have had no failure in this entire series. When treatment has been completed at the end of three to six months, we find that the range of motion is normal and foot function is normal.

Metatarsus Adductus

Metatarsus adductus, sometimes called metatarsus varus, can be best described as being one-third of a clubfoot since it is closely related to the adduction deformity found in every true case of clubfoot. The primary diagnostic factor here is the deviation of the forefoot towards the mid-line of the body at rest and on weight bearing. While the normal foot of a young child can be turned laterally at the mid-tarsus from ten to fifteen degrees, this foot resists all lateral movement and the lateral margin of the foot becomes convex in outline. The X-ray substantiates this finding but shows no rear foot involvement such as is found in the true clubfoot. If correction is not obtained, continued use in this abnormal position may lead to an inversion deformity and finally an equinus deformity which would eventually have to be treated as a true clubfoot. The idea that many children outgrow this condition or other deviations from the normal is absurd. Where certain children have been thought to outgrow them, they have never existed to any marked degree in the first place. That is also true of certain claims that such deformities have been corrected with strappings or shoe therapy. Such corrections were obtained with children who had borderline cases and the diagnosis was too severe.

The application of the skates to this problem again makes it almost certain, within human limitations, that correction will be achieved. For this problem the skates must be worn from four to six months in all, and some shoe therapy is required to maintain correction for a period of one to three years after the skates have been removed in the more aggravated conditions. After using the skates for that period, the foot will have motion at the midtarsus and the range of motion and foot function will be normal. In some instances, an exaggeration of medial rotation at the hip and a limitation of outward rotation will accompany this metatarsus adductus but that also will be corrected along with the foot problem.

According to our investigations, this is the first time in our profession that rotation abnormalities of the hip joints have been given any consideration with relation to problems of locomotion. We have become so intrigued with this subject and all of its ramifications that we wrote a paper on the anatomical and patho-mechanical manifestations associated with this rotation problem, especially in children. Our interest in this subject has led us to examine all adult patients for this condition; we have been confronted with some interesting findings.

There are many children who walk and stand with a decidedly abducted or adducted gait or stance and yet, when the feet are examined carefully, we find no pathology. When we check these children for rotation at the hip joints, we find that the deviations are often extreme. Where the normal limb of a child should be able to turn through an arc of 180 degrees—ninety degrees inward rotation and ninety degrees outward rotation, some of these children will have 180 degrees of motion distributed into thirty degrees inward rotation and 150 degrees outward rotation, or vice versa. In either case, therapy must be instituted before a fixation develops.

Our practices are filled with patients with severe foot problems due to this typical variation, and these same patients may be subject to arthritis of the knees, hips and spine as adults. The application of the skates to young children with this rotation abnormality brings about positive de-rotation and full correction within two to three months. At the end of this period of wear, the limbs will have a normal range of motion and the gait and stance of the patient will be within the normal range.

Cerebral Palsy

In the use of the skates for cerebral palsy children. Here we face the most trying and difficult task of treating of all foot and leg deformities in children. Paradoxically, there is no true structural deformity present until the child begins to use its locomotive structures and the abnormal use of these parts produces structural variations in the bones, joints and softer structures.

The basic pathological lesion in all cerebrals is in the brain or in the cerebellum and the tracts leading from the brain. It is an upper motor neuron lesion involving a destruction of brain and nerve tissue that cannot be repaired or replaced. Therefore, all treatment must be designed to utilize the remaining motor neuron structures in the training of affected muscles.

Cerebral victims received very little attention until 1930. As a consequence, there is very little literature available. Nevertheless every month brings new information related to the subject. Since there are five basic types of cerebral palsy recognized clinically and each of these types presents distinct variations in diagnosis and treatment, this subject will be covered more adequately in another chapter. In working with cerebrals, we have been able to make some observations of importance pertaining to our interests in the related foot and locomotive problems. Like all major problems that face the medical professions, the cerebral patients vary in severity from the mild to the most severe. We have found that skate therapy can be most beneficial for all but the most severe types where the victims are unable to control the muscles of the spine and head. Whenever these children can make some effort at standing and walking even with aid, the skates can become a most valuable adjunct to treatment. This is especially true of the types known as athetoids and the true spastics.

There are two basic reasons why the skates aid in the rehabilitation of these children:

1. The use of the skates limits and actually prevents the choreic or chaotic movements of these children because of their loss or impairment of the proprioceptive sense.

2. The use of the skates with the fixed range of motion within normal limits gives the child an opportunity to develop new neuromuscular pathways for simple locomotive activities.

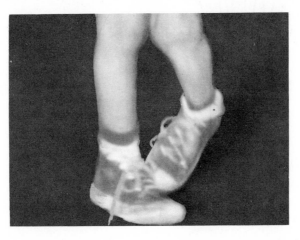

Fig. 57. Scissor's Gait—Young Child with Cerebral Palsy—Quadriplegic.

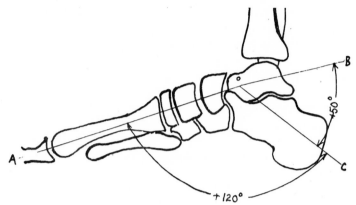

AXES AND ANGLES IN THE NORMAL FOOT. O: AXIAL CENTER. B: AXIS OF ASTRAGALUS
(TALUS) A: AXIS OF FIRST METATARSAL. C: AXIS OF CALCANEUS. THE AXES ARE DETERMINED
AS FOLLOWS: A ROENTGENOGRAM IS MADE, WITH THE LATERAL SURFACE OF THE FOOT RESTING
UPON THE CASSETTE. LINES ARE THEN DRAWN, (1) BISECTING THE FIRST METATARSAL, (2) FROM
THE TIP OF THE POSTERIOR TUBERCLE OF THE CALCANEUS THROUGH THE DEEPEST POINT ON THE
CALCANEAL SURFACE OF THE SINUS TARSI, AND (3) FROM THE POSTERIOR BORDER OF THE UPPER
ARTICULAR SURFACE OF THE TALUS THROUGH THE CENTER OF THE HEAD OF THAT BONE. NOTE THE
NORMAL CONTOUR OF THE CALCANEUS AND TALUS. (JOURNAL OF BONE & JOINT SURGERY: VOL. 28,
NO. 4, OCTOBER 1946)

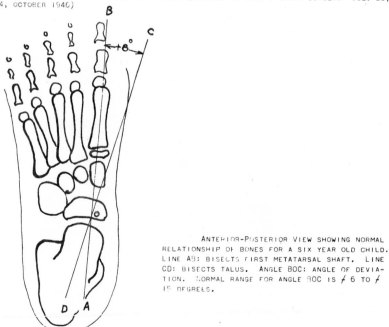

ANTERIOR-POSTERIOR VIEW SHOWING NORMAL
RELATIONSHIP OF BONES FOR A SIX YEAR OLD CHILD.
LINE AB: BISECTS FIRST METATARSAL SHAFT. LINE
CD: BISECTS TALUS. ANGLE BOC: ANGLE OF DEVIA-
TION. NORMAL RANGE FOR ANGLE BOC IS ∤ 6 TO ∤
15 DEGREES.

Fig. 58. Schematic Drawings Depicting X-rays of Normal Foot.

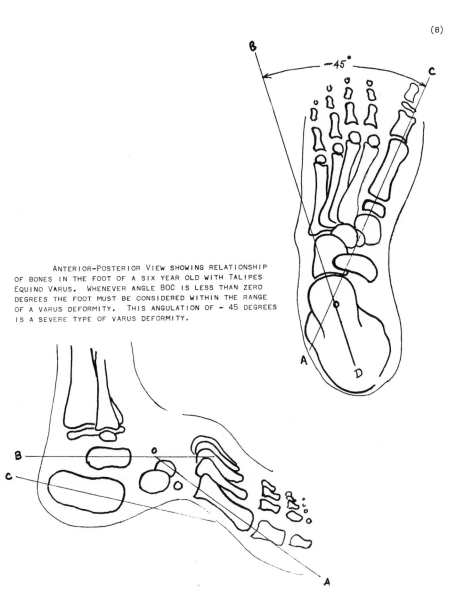

ANTERIOR-POSTERIOR VIEW SHOWING RELATIONSHIP
OF BONES IN THE FOOT OF A SIX YEAR OLD WITH TALIPES
EQUINO VARUS. WHENEVER ANGLE BOC IS LESS THAN ZERO
DEGREES THE FOOT MUST BE CONSIDERED WITHIN THE RANGE
OF A VARUS DEFORMITY. THIS ANGULATION OF - 45 DEGREES
IS A SEVERE TYPE OF VARUS DEFORMITY.

MEDIAL-LATERAL VIEW SHOWING RELATIONSHIP OF THE BONES IN SAME FOOT AS FIG. 3.
COMPARE WITH FIG. I AND OBSERVE ABNORMALITY HERE PRESENT. NOTE ALSO THE BLOCK TYPE
FORMATION OF THE TALUS AND CALCANEUS AS COMPARED WITH FIG. I.

Fig. 59. Schematic Drawings Depicting X-rays of Varus or Club Feet.

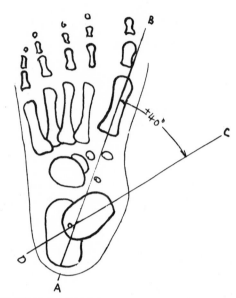

ANTERIOR-POSTERIOR VIEW SHOWING THE RELATIONSHIP OF BONES IN A CHILD OF SIX WITH A CALCANEO VALGUS TYPE FOOT. WHENEVER ANGLE BOC IS GREATER THAN ∠ 25 DEGREES, WE MUST CONSIDER THE FOOT IN THE RANGE OF VALGUS DEFORMITY. THIS ANGULATION OF ∠ 40 DEGREES IS A MODERATE-SEVERE TYPE OF VALGUS DEFORMITY.

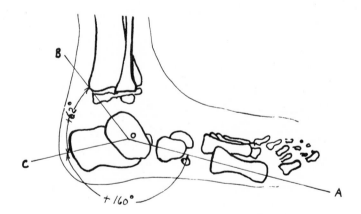

MEDIAL-LATERAL VIEW OF SAME FOOT AS FIG. 5. NOTE THE ANGULATION OF THE TALUS AS COMPARED WITH NORMAL IN FIG. 1. ALSO OBSERVE INCREASE OF ANGLE BC AND INCREASE OF ANGLE AC.

Fig. 60. Schematic Drawings Depicting X-rays of Valgus Feet.

15. TALIPES

Clubfoot is generally referred to as the congenital condition of the foot which produces an ankle type of walking. The word "talipes" is descriptive of this type of locomotion, because it is derived from the words "talus" meaning ankle and "pes" meaning foot. The most common type of deformity is the equinovarus type. In the "equinus" deformity the patient walks with the forefoot pointed downward and on the toes. The "varus" is descriptive of the inward turning of the foot on the leg.

While talipes equinovarus is the most common by far of all types of clubfoot, including both unilateral and bilateral, there are other congenital types of talipes which are more rare. These may be classified as:

1. Talipes equinovalgus
   In this condition the foot is rotated outward on the leg
2. Talipes calcaneovarus
   This deformity presents the heel in contact with the walking surface and the forefoot pointed upward.
3. Talipes calcaneovalgus
   Similar to the one above, except for the outward rotation of the foot on the leg.

Kite contends that the term clubfoot should be restricted to the talipes eqinovarus type of deformity. This deformity comprises ninety-five per cent of all of the cases in his experience, varying from the most severe to the mild types.

Other authorities prefer to call clubfoot "arthrogryposis multiplex congenita." The word "arthrogryposis" is derived from the Greek and means "curved joint."

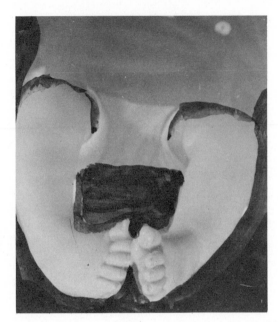

Fig. 61. Bilateral Talipes Equinovarus—Young Male.

Etiology

The predisposing factors in clubfoot appear to be hereditary with a family history of other congenital deformities. Kite has a series of statistics pointing out these factors. His figures show that twenty-two per cent of a series of cases under his observation gave a history of other members of the family having had clubfoot. The tendency was distributed through both parents. In thirteen per cent of the cases the brother or sister had clubfoot. Twelve per cent of the cases showed some other congenital deformity. In the series of 200 cases, sixty-seven and five tenths per cent were males and thiry-two and five tenths per cent females. Forty-six per cent were unilateral and fifty-four per cent bilateral. In the unilateral cases the right foot was involved forty-three per cent and the left fifty-seven per cent.

Most present-day authorities do not advance the theory that clubfoot is caused by intra-uterine pressure or abnormal position. The fact remains that no positive proof has yet been obtained concerning the factors causing clubfoot.

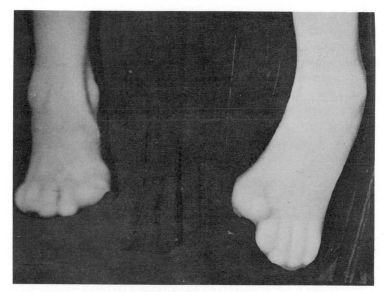

Fig. 62. Unilateral Talipes Equinovarus.

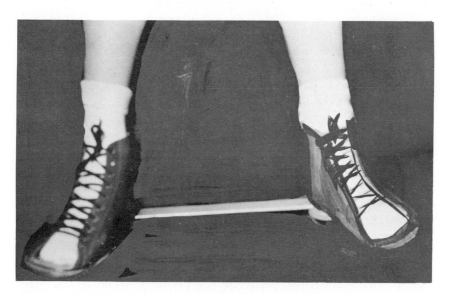

Fig. 63. Figure 62 with Skates Holding Feet in Correction.

Pathology

Since there are three component parts to the involvement of club-foot, each of these should be considered separately:

1. There is adduction of the forefoot far beyond the normal range of motion.
2. There is an inversion of the foot which is also beyond the normal range of motion.
3. There is the equinus deformity in which plantar flexion is greatly exaggerated. The adduction deformity may be mild to very extreme.

At birth the relationship of the foot to the leg may be a complete reversal from the normal and in such a deformity the toes may actually be in the same position as the heel of the normal foot. This motion takes place primarily in the talonavicular articulation and in the calcaneo-cuboid joints. Inversion or the inward turning of the foot occurs primarily in the talocalcaneal and talonavicular articulations. The equinus deformity takes place in the talonavicular and calcaneocuboid joints. The under-standing of the function of the feet and the muscles of the leg controlling the action of the feet makes it clear that all of the contracted muscles which control the motion of the joints will become stronger and the stretched muscles will become weakened. As the child develops and the bones of the foot are allowed to remain in abnormal apposition to each other, these structures become adjusted to their malposition and the de-formity becomes more and more fixed.

If no correction is instituted before the child begins to walk, the distortion becomes more and more aggravated. For that reason most authorities advocate treatment from the first day of birth.

The author believes that not enough attention has been given to the relationship between the clubfoot and the unequalized muscular ten-sion of the inward rotators of the thigh. It will be observed that the abnormal relationship of the two groups of muscles in the foot or leg, such as the abductors and adductors or the supinators and pronators, will produce definite secondary changes in the muscles of the thigh. It can also be observed that in most instances of talipes equinovarus the ad-ductors or inward rotators of the thigh are far too powerful in their ac-tion, and the abductors or outward rotators are weak by comparison. While normal relationship of these two groups would be approximately two to one, where talipes exists the relationship is far in excess of that ratio. Thus, it is the author's contention that the inward rotation of the

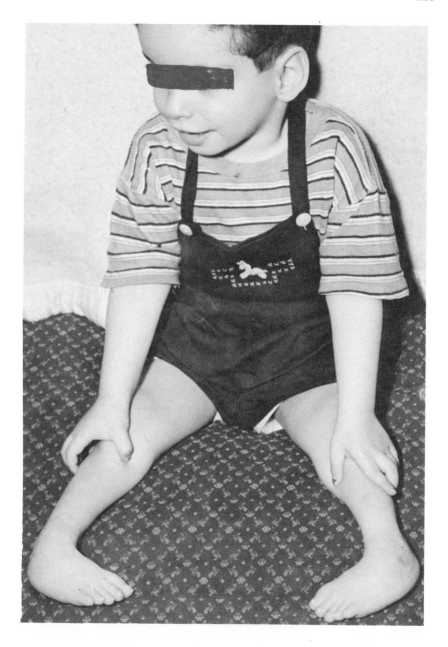

Fig. 64. Two Year Old Male with Severe Talipes Equinovarus.

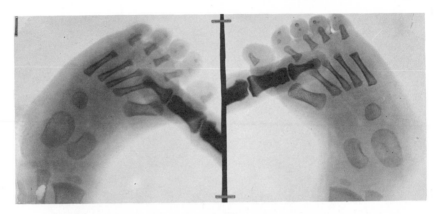

Fig. 65. X-rays of Patient in Fig. 64 at Six Months of Age.

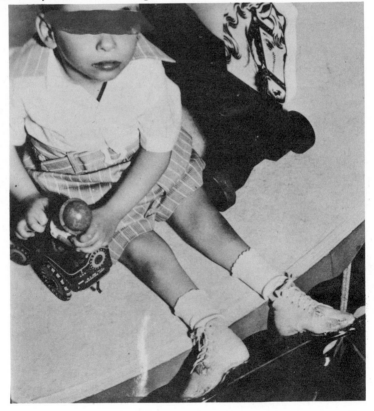

Fig. 66. Same Patient with Skates Applied in Correction.

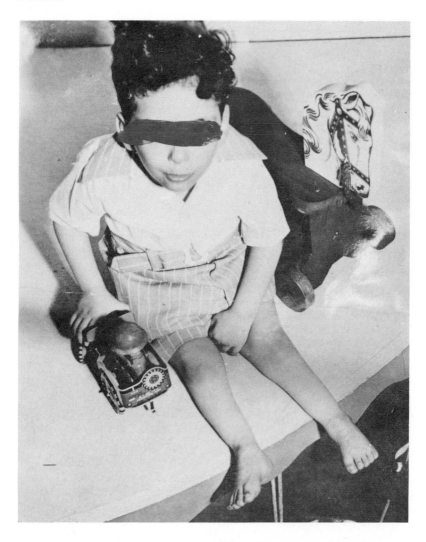

Fig. 67. Same Patient after Six Months of Treatment with Skates.

thighs must be controlled for proper correction of talipes equinovarus, especially when weight bearing has started.

Diagnosis

Since true talipes equinovarus and the other more rare club-foot deformities are present at birth, the diagnosis is relatively simple. Acquired clubfoot deformities can occur as a result of a number of diseases, including Friedreich's ataxia, scarlet fever, poliomyelitis, muscular involvements, fractures and many debilitating diseases of childhood. Deformities simulating clubfoot can also occur in later life as a result of disturbances affecting the nerve center of the body.

Prognosis

For many years the classical treatment of clubfoot, which included plaster of paris casting, forcible manipulation and surgery, produced variable results. The prognosis, therefore, was always dependent upon a large variety of factors and could never be determined with true accuracy. At best, the child born with a talipes condition was almost doomed to some type of deformity in spite of all efforts.

Treatment

Since the classical treatment for talipes equinovarus has been plaster of paris casting, forcible manipulation and surgery. Along with this, the simple home care of massage and mild manipulation was usually instituted. Most authorities advocated that the treatment should begin very early, preferably from the first week of birth. During the first few weeks the treatment usually consisted of strapping, massage, and manipulations. In these treatments all three deformities, the varus, the equinus, and supination were dealt with as much as possible.

As the infant grew older, depending upon its physical progress, plaster of paris casts were applied anywhere from the second week after birth in a normal, healthy child, up to the third month in an underdeveloped child. New casts were applied every three to four weeks and with each new application the foot was placed in a more severe over-corrected position. This therapy was usually continued for a period of three months to one year or until such time as other factors interfered with the continual application of casts.

When the casting technique was considered sufficient, the child was allowed to remain without casts for a short period of time to determine whether or not the deformity would recur. In the meantime, massage and manipulation was continued. In most instances a recurrence did take

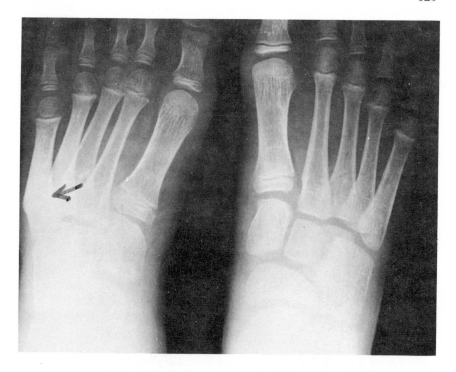

Fig. 68. Stress Fracture of Fifth Metatarsal Brace Occurring Three Years after Correction and Resulting from Inadequate Aftercare.

place. One of the primary factors pertaining to clubfoot is the ease with which the foot returns to its abnormal relationship with the leg.

The next steps in treatment were usually a return to plaster of paris casting for another extended period of time, or surgery. The surgical correction varied in its technique and depended upon various factors. In some instances surgery brought about fair cosmetic results, but poor functional results. The steps in the treatment outlined above were usually continued from infancy to the adult period of life.

The author is stressing the great variation in techniques employed because it is his belief that the entire field of clubfoot treatment must be reviewed and approached from the mechanical standpoint so that both good functional and cosmetic results may be obtained. There are too many patients who could have been saved the many difficulties they encountered in their treatment of clubfoot had such a study been instituted long ago.

One of the disagreeable effects of the cast therapy can be found in the unilateral type, especially where the application of casts prevented the normal development of the affected extremity while the opposite extremity was growing. Thus, we have these victims with not only a clubfoot, but a shortened and weakened extremity also.

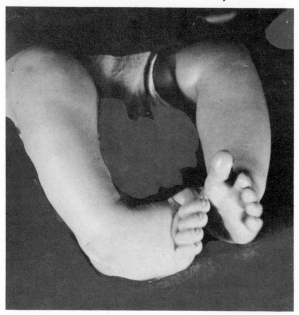

Fig. 69. Severe Talipes Equinovarus in Young Child.

Case Report—Talipes Equinovarus

In 1946, when Kenneth M. was one year old, his parents brought him to our office for consultation. Kenneth was born with a talipes equinovarus of the left foot and for a period of eight months he was in and out of plaster-of-paris casts with apparently little or no success in correcting the condition. When surgery was advised, the parents decided to continue conservative methods of treatment before acquiescing.

Kenneth was a normal, healthy child in every respect except for the deformed foot. There was a slight impairment of the muscle structure of the left leg but the condition could not be classified as severe. All ranges

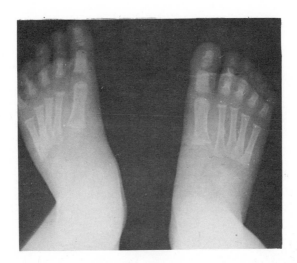

Fig. 70. Dorso-plantar X-ray Views of Patient K. M.—Two Years Old.

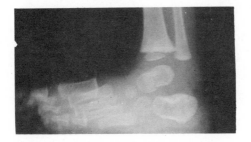

Fig. 71. Same Patient—Left Foot—Medial Lateral View.

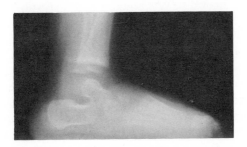

Fig. 72. Same Patient—Right Foot—Medial Lateral View.

of motion above the ankle were quite normal. The only restriction appeared to be in the foot and ankle. Since the child was just beginning to stand up on his feet and had not yet initiated walking, the parents were advised to use our skates for a period of twenty-four hours a day and to remove them only when the child was being dressed and bathed. This program was continued for a period of six months without variation. During this time, Kenneth learned how to stand and walk with the skates. He was a very active child and there was little restriction in his movements because of the skates.

At the end of six months, he was allowed to go without the skates for a period of six hours a day for the following six months. When he was two years of age, the skates were removed as a daytime measure and they were only used at night. At thirty months of age the skates were removed completely.

For walking purposes, the parents were instructed to obtain high keds and the entire outer margin of the left ked was wedged from heel to toe to a thickness of 1/4″. Kenneth was kept in keds and this wedging was continued until the boy was twelve years old.

We saw Kenneth approximately every four to six months during this period of time and serial X-rays were taken from time to time to make certain that the clubfoot did not recur.

After the boy approached puberty he was allowed to obtain normal shoes and we fitted him with a balance inlay that had the lateral margin wedged to approximately 1/8″. The left foot was approximately one size shorter than the right foot, but again the balance inlay compensated for the difference in size. The balance inlays were changed approximately every two years as he outgrew them. Kenneth developed into a tall, strapping boy with a considerable amount of athletic ability. In his senior year of high school, he became captain of the golf team and won an athletic scholarship to a college where he continued to play golf and became captain of his college team.

In observing Kenneth at the present time, there is no indication that he ever had any problem with his foot, but a close examination of the foot will reveal some deformity was present. He has some mild fatigue on the left side after strenuous activity. We believe that if he will continue to wear balance inlays he will be able to go through life without any apparent further difficulty.

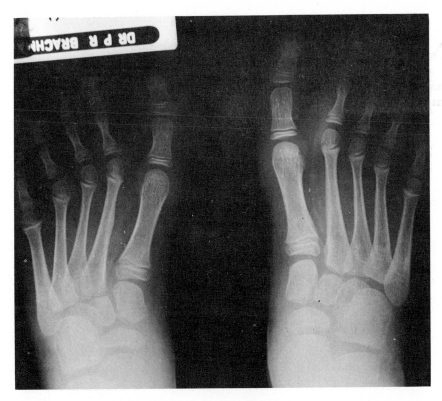

Fig. 73. Patient K. M. at Sixteen Years of Age.

Case History—Talipes Equinovalgus

Some of the more severe foot problems in infants and children re-spond well to mechanical therapy if the problem to be resolved can be attended to without any relapse in treatment over a period of years. In most instances this means that the problem has to be treated until the primary growth factors in the foot and leg have been attained, at least through puberty. In many instances the patients require additional treatment after they have reached puberty and into their adult years. Several case histories will be listed here that may bear out these findings.

In 1946 Roco R., five years of age, was brought to our office with a history of birth deformity to his left foot and leg. On several occasions since birth the child had been treated by casting, but the parents had not allowed any single doctor to complete his course of treatment because they contended that everyone they had gone to wanted to perform surgery and they had decided that surgery was out of the question.

Upon examination it was found that the boy had a typical talipes equinovalgus. The X-rays confirmed this diagnosis and also revealed a marked plantar talus in association with the deformity. All normal ranges of motion were absent and muscular power was deficient in all muscles that entered the foot from the leg. The leg was atrophied below the knee and there appeared to be a shortage of approximately 3/4" in the limb itself in comparison with the right limb.

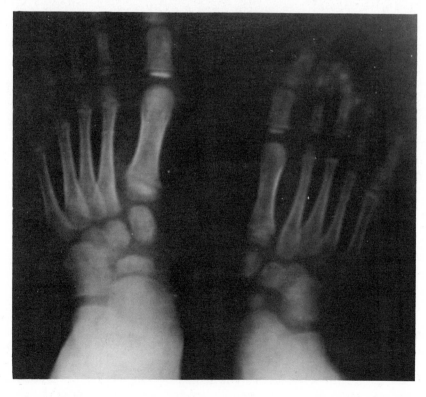

Fig. 74. Patient Roco R.—Dorso-plantar View at Age Fourteen.

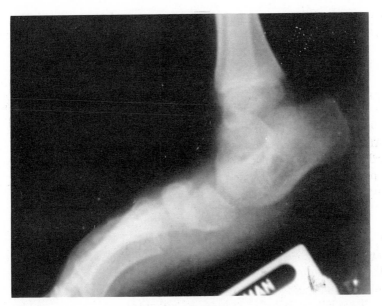

Fig. 75. Patient Roco R.—Medial Lateral View—Note Plantar Talus.

Associated with this problem was a rotational deformity of the entire limb at the hip. The limb could be rotated outward to approximately ninety degrees but inward rotation was limited to zero. Consequently, the boy walked with a marked abducted outward-rotated gait and the parents advised us that he became fatigued quite readily. It was evident from the start that it would be necessary to bring about as much internal rotation as possible and that we would have to try to maintain a more normal relationship between the foot and the ankle before much change could be achieved in the boy's gait and posture.

Accordingly, we instituted a series of manipulative treatments and decided to use our ambulatory skate devices to correct the de-rotation and abduction of the foot and leg. We instructed the parents in the use of the skates and advised them that they were to be worn for twenty hours out of every twenty-four. There was no correction applied to the left foot but the right foot was held in such a position that no external rotation was permitted. Only internal rotation could be achieved if the child had any desire to walk. At the same time we saw the child once each week for manipulation and we also advised the parents how to manipulate the child's foot every day for a period of ten to fifteen minutes.

After two months there was sufficient internal rotation to eliminate the use of the skates during the daytime, and the parents were advised to apply them only for night wear. At the same time manipulation had achieved some of the results we anticipated and we constructed a stainless steel Roberts plate for the left foot.

After six months the skates were no longer necessary because full inward rotation had been achieved and the direction of the child's walk with his right foot was comparable to that of the normal left foot. At this point manipulation was also discontinued. The parents were instructed to bring the boy back every three months and were advised that it would be necessary to continue the use of the Roberts plate for an indefinite period of time, possibly for years.

During the following twenty years, as the boy grew into adulthood, we saw him approximately ten to twelve times. As each plate was outgrown or worn out, they were replaced. This continued until two years ago when we decided to substitute a balance inlay for Roberts plate because Rocco had been working as a draftsman for several years and was no longer on his feet as much as he was when he was younger. The balance inlays served two purposes: since the left foot was approximately two sizes shorter than the right, it filled the unused space in the shoe without making it necessary for him to obtain split sizes; also, it gave him a considerable sense of relief when he was on his feet. From all appearances at this time, Rocco will have a good-functioning foot for the remainder of his life.

Talipes Equinovalgus—A Case Report

Michael S. was nineteen months old when he was first brought to our office. He was born with a bilateral talipes equinovalgus, and when he was five days old, casts were applied to both feet and legs. These casts were changed at three-to four-week intervals for a period of nine months. From the ninth month to the nineteenth month, the physician in charge of his treatment used various shoe modalities and/or corrective methods of choice. An examination of Michael revealed there was no motion whatever at the mid-tarsus. Both feet had "rocker bottoms" and there was no flexion or extension at the ankle joint unless the foot was held in marked abduction. Michael's legs were fairly well developed and there did not appear to be any disability in the muscular structure itself in either limb. Both the right and the left limbs could be rotated

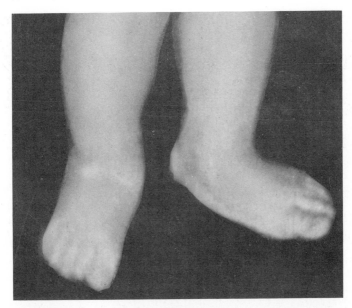

Fig. 76. Michael S.—Age 18 Months—Talipes Equinovalgus.

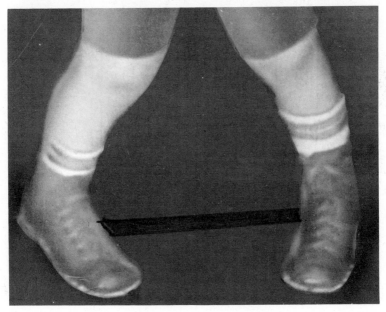

Fig. 77. Michael S. Wearing Shoes with "Skates" Set for Correction.

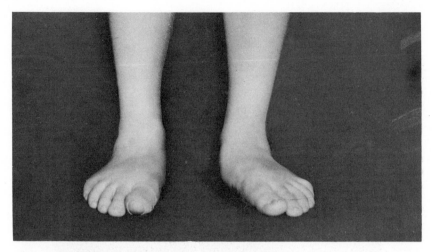

Fig. 78. Michael S. After Two Years of Treatment.

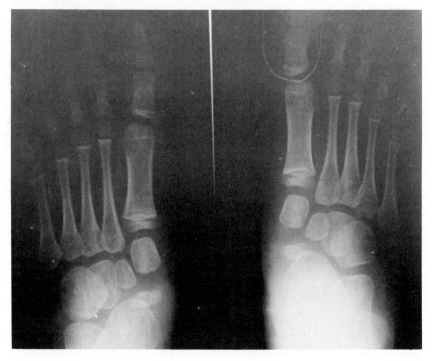

Fig. 79. Michael S.—Dorso-Plantar Views at Four Years of Age.

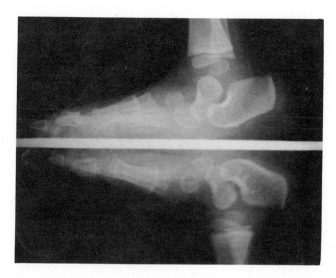

Fig. 80. Michael S.—Medial-Lateral Views at 18 Months.

outward to the point where the toes and the heels were reversed in position. This amounted to approximately 180° of outward rotation. There was no inward rotation possible with either limb.

Anterior-posterior and medial-lateral X-ray views demonstrated the severity of the plantar talus bilaterally and showed the typical changes that one finds present in a talipes equinovalgus. The child walked with both limbs rotated in a marked outward position and both feet bore weight on the inner aspects of the feet with the brunt of the weight falling on the medial posterior aspects of the calcaneus and the talonavicular articulation. As a consequence, the gait was labored and ungainly. The parents informed us that the child was not steady on his feet and fell quite often.

Michael was fitted with ambulatory skates attached to the shoes and he wore these for a period of twenty-two hours a day for one year. The skates were set in such a position that he could not rotate his limbs or his feet outward at any time. Every few months, the position was changed so that he had to use the skates set in a position of inward rotation. He learned how to walk with these after several days and from that time on he had no difficulty in ambulation with the devices.

At the end of one year, Michael continued to use the skates for six hours during the day and for full night-time wear. He was also fitted with a pair of Roberts plates at this stage and they were placed in the shoes he wore when not using the skates.

At the end of one year, Michael continued to use the skates for longer used the skates for day-time wear, but they were continued for night wear only. An examination demonstrated a normal range of inward and outward rotation at the hip joints and that his motion at the ankle joint in the range of flexion, extension, abduction and adduction were almost within normal limits.

Follow-up X-rays taken every six months, revealed the changes that had taken place. We also took motion pictures of Michael's progress from the time the treatment was initiated. At the end of the second year, the skates were discontinued entirely and the boy was still wearing the Roberts plates. From the second to the fifth year of treatment new Roberts plates were applied as Michael outgrew the old ones and there was no recurrence of the talipes equinovalgus.

This child was followed for several years afterward. He attended school and kept up at the same pace with other boys of his own age without any complaints. We continued to take X-rays about once each year and examination of Michael's feet when he was eight years old revealed that he had a marked pes planus type of foot with very little valgus present, and the plantar talus which was present at an early age was still in evidence but not to such a marked degree. Since the rocker bottom had been eliminated, the plantar talus did not cause any deformity on weight bearing. Michael's case is another good example of the value of mechanical therapy in the long term treatment of these congenital deformities.

Talipes Equinovarus—A Case Report

Jeffery H. was brought to our office when he was two years and ten months old. Since birth he had been treated for talipes equinovarus of the right foot. The left foot was normal. From birth until eight months of age the foot was treated with plaster of paris splints which were replaced approximately every four weeks. There was no significant improvement of the foot at the end of that period. For an additional period of approximately one year, Jeffery was treated with Denis-Browne splints at night and with his shoes wedged along the outer margin for daytime wear. Again there was no significant improvement.

Prior to coming to our office, the surgeon who had been attending Jeffery was prepared to do a rotation osteotomy but the parents would not agree to this type of surgery.

Examination of Jeffery revealed that there was a marked limitation of motion at the ankle joint in the range of dorsiflexion, with about fifteen degrees of plantar flexion. The foot was held in a fixed inverted and adducted position. Subjectively, Jeffrey could not dorsiflex his foot or evert it to the slightest degree. The anterior and posterior tibials were strong as were the gastrocnemius and soleus. Jeffery walked with a typical talipes equinovarus gait and bore weight on the outer and lateral margins of his foot. There was a prominent area of weight bearing at the base of the fifth metatarsal and a considerable bursa had already developed at this area. Associated with this problem, Jeffrey also had a marked limitation of outward rotation at the hip joint with an inward rotation of approximately 140 degrees.

Anterior-posterior and medial-lateral X-rays were taken and all X-ray findings were typical of talipes equinovarus of a severe degree.

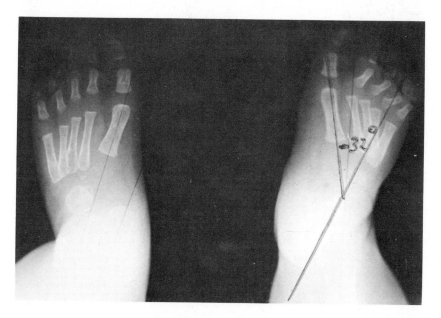

Fig. 81. Jeffrey H.—Two Years Old—Dorso-Plantar Views of Unilateral Talipes Equinovarus.

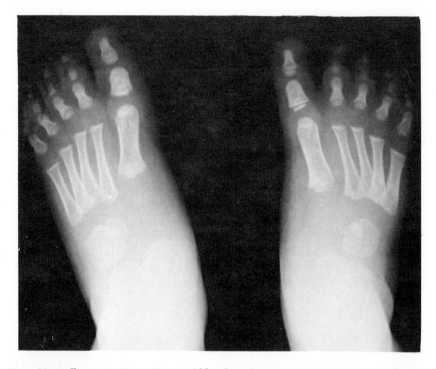

Fig. 82. Jeffrey H.—Four Years Old after Treatment for Two Years with "Skates.

The parents agreed to cooperate fully in the use of the ambulatory skates. They were requested to apply the skates for the entire walking period with the exception of two hours a day, and then to apply them again for nightwear. This program was continued for a period of six months. At the end of the first month, dramatic improvement in some of the ranges of motion were noted. By the sixth month, the foot could be dorsiflexed and abducted at the midtarsus and ankle joint with considerable ease. Jeffery had no problems wearing the skates during the hours specified. However, when the skates were removed at the end of six months, Jeffery's gait was not completely normal. There was a considerable amount of improvement in his walking, but still a tendency toward some adduction and inversion on weightbearing. At this stage, Jeffrey was fitted with a metal Roberts plate and the parents were asked to obtain high keds with the instructions that the entire outer

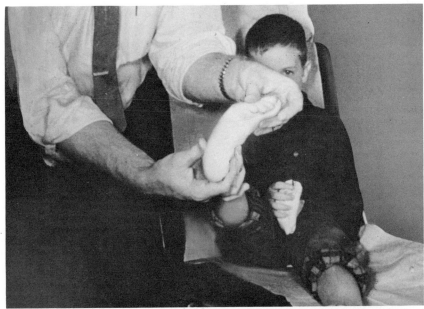

Fig. 83. Jeffrey H. at Six Years, Demonstrating Limits of Foot Inversion.

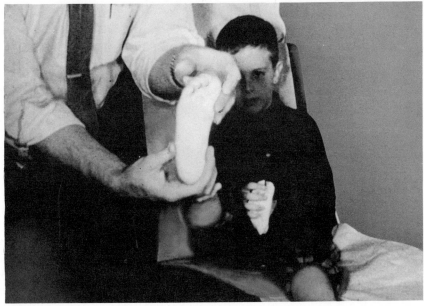

Fig. 84. Jeffrey H.—Demonstrating Normal Alignment of Foot.

sole area was to be wedged on the outside approximately three-eighths inch. They were also instructed to have Jeffrey wear these skates for one-half of his waking hours and to continue them for full-time nightwear. This program was continued for an additional six months. At the end of one year, considerable additional improvement was noted, and the use of the skates as a daytime measure was discontinued. At this stage, with the metal plate in the shoe that was wedged on the outer sole area, and Jeffrey was asked to walk barefooted, the right foot did go into a symptoms while the shoe was being worn. When the shoe was removed and Jeffery was asked to walk bare-footed, the right foot did go into a varus and adducted position to some degree.

We decided to construct a plantar appliance out of plastic material which contained the entire plantar surface of the foot and literally hooked around the first metatarsal-phalangeal segment. After wearing this appliance in the keds for several months, it was observed that Jeffrey could abduct the forefoot subjectively against gravity. The parents were instructed to give the child resistance exercises in the range of abduction and dorsiflexion. These exercises were given every night when possible and continued for a period of approximately one year. In the meantime, Jeffrey wore the plastic device and had a second one made when he outgrew the first.

At the present time after approximately three years of treatment, Jeffrey has unusually good results from the mechanical therapy employed. Despite the fact that these results have been good, we will continue to see Jeffery every 3 to 6 months until puberty and he will continue to wear these Keds with wedged sole for an additional six to seven years.

This type of follow-up treatment is very essential in conditions of talipes equinovarus because of the great tendency for the problem to recur.

16. RETARDED BONY DEVELOPMENT OF MID-TARSUS

It has been more than 25 years since we first described the clinical findings in the conditions that we termed the osseous retardation of the mid-tarsus in children. Since that time we have amassed a large number of X-rays of children's feet, between the ages of 4 and 7, which demonstrate this marked retardation in the development of the navicular, alone and in some instances, the middle and medial cuneiforms and the heads of the lesser metatarsals.

Symptomatically, these children complain of early fatigue, and the parents always state that the child refuses to walk any distances but wants to be carried. These are also the children who complain of vague foot and leg pains during the night. There are no positive symptomatic findings on subjective examination and the objective findings are not outstanding in most instances. The ranges of motion are not usually abnormal and muscles do not demonstrate any noticeable weakness.

The only consistent physical finding is a rather low arched foot with some pronation present. But even that is not excessive. It is only after an X-ray has been taken that we can make a positive diagnosis. In some instances, the X-ray will reveal rudimentary areas of ossification for some of the midtarsal bones and on occasion one foot will reveal a more rapid type of ossification than the other. When the navicular bone alone is involved, it almost appears in some instances that Kohler's osteochondritis is present. However, the symptoms of pain and all other factors associated with Kohler's is never found, and the confusion of Kohler's disease with the condition must be avoided.

145

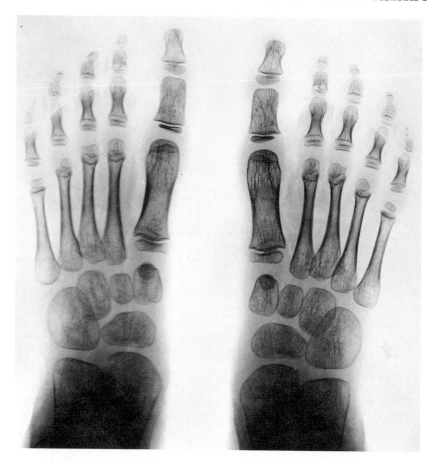

Fig. 85. Dorso-Plantar X-rays—Normal Bony Development and Alignment for Six Year Old Female.

    This type of retarded development of the midtarsal bones can often be found in several children of the same family so it is possible that familiar tendency may be involved and it may be said to be genetic. It must be understood that no vacuum exists in the midtarsal area because the bones do not show up as radiopaque substances on X-ray. We are dealing with embryonic structures which have not yet had the opportunity to ossify and we feel that our greatest problem is associated with

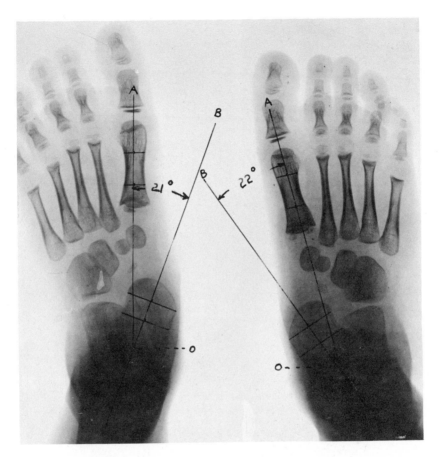

Fig. 86. Dorso-Plantar X-rays—Retarded Development of Naviculars in Six
Year Old Female, with Associated Deviation of Tali.

the attachments of the posterior tibial muscle and to some extent, the
anterior tibial, to the navicular and its surrounding structures. If there
is no true basic solid substance for this attachment, we must reason
that the function of the tibial muscles cannot be carried out adequately
and consequently there must be some sagging of the foot at the mid-
tarsal area. Since the tarsus has been shown to be one of the primary
areas where weakness can occur on weight bearing, we must come
to the aid of these structures when we find bony retardation present.

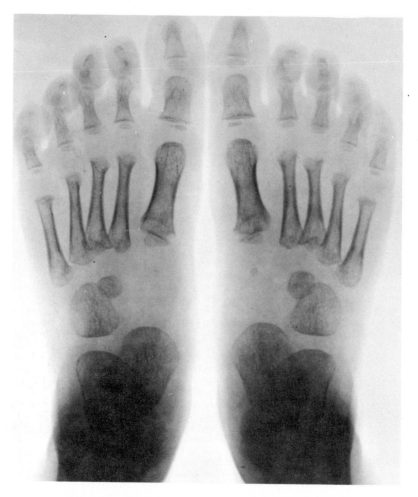

Fig. 87. Dorso-Plantar X-rays—Retarded Mid-Tarsal Development in Five
     Year Old Male.

It has been our opinion that mechanical support, with the help of
proper food supplements, will bring about the proper bony development
of the mid-tarsal bones of the foot within a relatively short period of
time to prevent complete breakdown. For these conditions, we prefer
the use of metal therapy which is discussed in another chapter.

Meade discusses the problem of juvenile pes plano-valgus. It is
his theory that a muscular imbalance between the medial and lateral

segments of the foot brings on this condition and he describes a metal appliance which cups the tarsal and midtarsal areas of the foot and extends forward under the shafts of the fourth and fifth metatarsals, designed to bring the foot back into its normal balanced relationship.

Thomson, in describing the treatment of congenital flatfoot, is particularly interested in the ease with which the dorsum of the foot can be placed against the leg itself so that the foot is held in the calcaneal valgus position against the leg. When the child crawls, the foot is also held in pronounced pronation and eversion. He asks why it is that otherwise healthy-looking, well-developed young men should be afflicted with poor feet, and he wonders whether or not it is reasonable to suggest that they had this condition at birth and also whether or not this condition would have been improved had their muscles been exercised during infancy and early childhood. In his comments at the close of his article, Thomson writes: "Faulty posture, instability and abnormal mobility are all aggravated by habit. When these characteristics are combined with congenital weakness of the infant foot, the condition must be corrected by the following means: proper muscular activity in the right, or over-corrected posture must be developed and new habits of the intrinsic foot muscles, as well as of the extrinsic leg muscles must be created."

In discussing a small group of controlled cases, Thomson states, "Most of these children, although still quite young, have pronated valgus feet and several are already symptomatic. A few however, have developed very normal feet. The question, of course, remains as to what will happen to these patients later in life. Since the congenital clubfoot is usually a foot with limited possibilities, many of the congenital flat feet which have been treated, although they. look normal, may maintain normal function."

An interesting comment appears at the close of the article, and relates to a simple procedure which has also been used in mild calcaneal valgus cases. In these cases, the soles of the infant's feet were held together with compound tincture of benzoin and bound with a two-inch elastic bandage. This position of the soles in the inverted position and held together was maintained for a period of three to four months. There appeared to be little or no objection to this method of treatment by the parents. In most instances this treatment seemed to have produced some adequate results. Because there has been no further follow-up of this treatment in the literature, it is difficult to determine what the results have been in long series of cases.

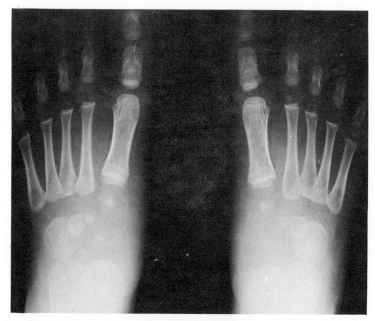

Fig. 88. Dorso-Plantar X-rays—Retarded Mid-Tarsal Development in Seven Year Old Male.

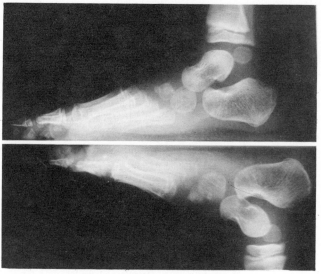

Fig. 89. Medial Lateral X-rays—Same Patient.

17. OSTEOCHONDRITIS

Freiberg's Disease

One of the common sites of osteochondritis in the foot is found in the second metatarsal head. This condition is often referred to as Freiberg's infraction or Freiberg's disease. Originally it was described pathologically as a disease that affects the second metatarsal-phalangeal joint, and sometimes may be found in the third. Freiberg believed that injury was the most prominent etiological factor. Since some of his patients were able to trace the original injury to active play on the tennis courts, he felt that the trauma received to the second metatarsal head during the game of tennis caused the problem. Many other orthopedic surgeons held the same view as Freiberg and the etiology became established with them in the term of an eggshell fracture and associated with younger people who played tennis.

This etiology, however, fails to explain the osteochondritis that develops in the second metatarsal head of some young children between the ages of four and ten. In most instances all of the cardinal signs of inflammation are present and the area is quite painful. The pain lasts approximately two weeks and, after that healing takes place almost spontaneously but usually leaves a wide and flattened metatarsal head which may or may not cause considerable problems as time goes on because the second metatarsal head is a major factor in weight bearing and if it extends beyond the first head, it will bear more than its normal share of weight.

Kohler's Disease

Kohler reported the same condition very shortly after Freiberg. Kohler does not believe that trauma plays the most important role

151

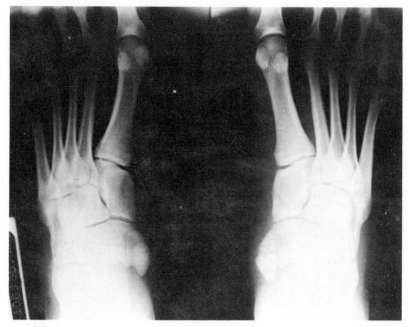

Fig. 90. X-ray Showing Supernumerary Naviculars. (Os Tibiale Externum).

in the development of this disease. He calls this condition a pathological entity of unknown origin. There is also some thought that the
condition is present because of the interference of essential nutritional
factors in the second or third metatarsal shaft and head.

Since there is only one foramen in each metatarsal shaft through
which a plantar blood vessel may enter the shaft of the bone and the
head for nutritional purposes, if that artery is injured or interfered
with, there is certain to be a necrosis of the bone or at least some interference in the development of the head of that shaft. Whatever the
etiological factor may be, there is epiphyseal bone cartilage degeneration,
and the problem does require attention when it exists.

While the chief symptom is usually pain, there is also restriction of
joint motion and a crepitation may be felt in the joint on dorsiflexion
and plantar flexion. There is localized tenderness surrounding the
joint with thickening and swelling of the surrounding structures. The
patient cannot walk directly on the forefoot and usually bears weight
on the heel while the pain lasts. Radiographically, the head of the sec-

ond metatarsal bone shows destruction and the normal rounded appearance of the head is lost. The margin of the bone is rough and irregular and after healing takes place, the end of the bone is widened and thickened along its entire articular margin and the adjoining phalanx may also be widened and thickened to correspond with the metatarsal head.

During the acute stage it may be possible to relieve the pain and improve weight bearing by proper strapping with plaster of paris and padding of the involved area so as to remove weight bearing from the second or third metatarsal head. A Thomas bar placed on the sole of the shoe may also bring some additional relief. Where there is considerable pain involved, it is best to have the patient remain off weight bearing for approximately two weeks' time. There are times when plaster of paris casts applied to the foot will bring the necessary relief.

After the condition has healed, it is often necessary to perform surgery on this second metatarsal head and the approximating phalanx in order to bring about the maximum amount of comfort on weight bearing. One of our patients, a young, healthy, fourteen-year-old male, developed this condition at the second metatarsal head during his first year in high school. After the painful conditions had been eliminated, he was fitted with a full metal plantar plate, extending from the heel to the end of his toes because he could not bear weight properly without having constant pain whenever the second metatarsal-phalangeal articulation was dorsiflexed.

Since the metal plate prevented dorsiflexion of this joint, he was able to continue most of his activities without difficulty. In fact, he was quite active in athletics and wore this plate at all times until he had finished high school and college. After he had completed his college work and before he started his business career, we performed surgery on the foot and reconstructed the second metatarsal head and the adjacent phalanx. After the surgery was performed, it was no longer necessary for him to wear any type of appliance.

Osteochondritis of Navicular

The navicular bone in young children is also subject to osteochondrosis. A synonym for this disease is Kohler's disease of the navicular. The etiology is thought to be injury of some type, associated with an interference of the blood supply of the navicular. It appears that the ossification center of this bone is involved, resulting in retardation of its osseous development. On X-ray the bone appears to be fragmented and very dense in comparison with the surrounding bone tissue. The tissue in the area of the navicular is sensitive to movement and tender to pressure. The child will limp and prefers to bear weight on the outer border of the foot. In most instances all of the signs of inflammation are present and remain for a period of approximately two weeks.

The medial-lateral X-ray view of the foot shows the navicular in similar shape to that of a silver half-dollar standing on edge. Healing appears to be spontaneous but if the condition persists in causing pain and disability, the foot may be strapped with adhesive tape or a plaster-of paris cast applied to hold the foot in slight varus. Since this condition is usually found in children from three to seven or eight years of age and is primarily unilateral, the diagnosis is not too difficult to make. The osteochondritis causes a retardation in the development of the navicular bone and therefore, it is usually necessary to use supportive measures for a considerable time after the original treatment is rendered. We have found that the metal Whitman plate or the Roberts plate is best for this purpose.

Calcaneal Apophysitis

Osteochondritis of the epiphysis of the calcaneus has been described in the literature but this condition is not very common. It must not be confused with apophysitis of the calcaneus which is not truly an osteochondritis but rather an injury to the area of growth appearing in the cap of the calcaneus. In order to make a diagnosis of osteochondritis of the calcaneus or Sever's disease, it would be necessary to have all of the cardinal signs of inflammation present. When these are present, it is usually necessary for the child to refrain from bearing weight on the heel because the pain is too great. In most instances it is necessary to immobilize the foot to overcome this disability. We have seen numerous instances of apophysitis of the calcaneus but have never encountered a single instance of Sever's disease or osteochondritis of the calcaneus during our period of practice. It is entirely possible that this disease, or so-called disease, is truly non-existent.

We believe that the same statement can be made for osteochondritis of the base of the fifth metatarsal bone. Such a condition, or one that is described as osteochondritis, is possibly due to injury of the base of the fifth metatarsal bone where severe pain and an inflammatory process may set up. This would not be a true disease, but in fact an injury and should be treated as such under the designation of fracture.

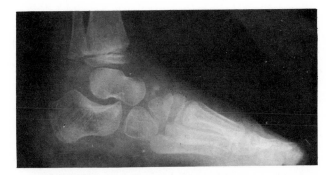

Fig. 91. X-ray of Six Year Old Female.

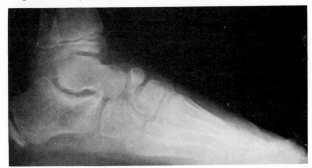

Fig. 92. X-ray of Same Patient at Eight Years, Showing Beginning of Calcaneal Cap. Note Abnormal Development of Navicular in this Talipes Equino Varus Foot.

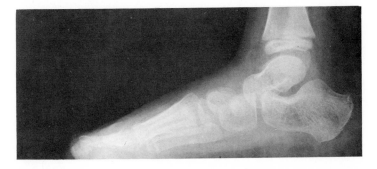

Fig. 93. X-ray of Nine Year Old Male—No Calcaneal Cap.

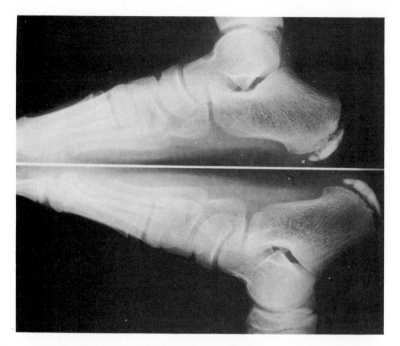

Fig. 94. X-ray of Twelve Year Old Male—Calcaneal Apophysitis.

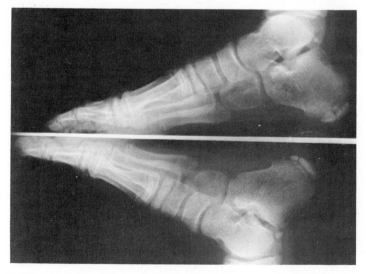

Fig. 95. X-ray of Nine Year Old Female—Calcaneal Apophysitis.

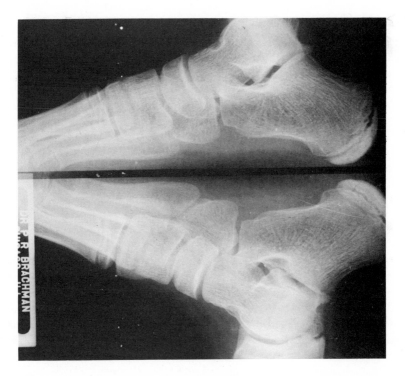

Fig. 96. X-ray of Thirteen Year Old Male—Normal Growth of Calcaneal Cap—
No Fragmentation.

Spastic Flatfoot

Harris and Beath have demonstrated that certain cases of peroneal
spastic flatfoot were caused by a medial talocalcaneal bridge, and at
the same time concurred in observations of Slomann and Badgley that
a calcaneo-navicular bar also accounted or peroneal spastic flatfoot.
Their final conclusion was that peroneal spastic flatfoot is a clinical
manifestation of a congenital tarsal fusion. The present retrospect is a
summarization of their knowledge based on a review of the records of
102 cases of spastic flatfoot. Since 91 of the 102 cases consisted of medial
talocalcaneal bridge and calcaneo-navicular bars, Harris suggested
that other bony fusions which brought on peroneal spastic flatfoot were
rather rare and less disabling and of academic rather than clinical importance.

The discussion in this article did not relate to peroneal spastic flatfoot which might be caused by other disabilities such as arthritis and traumatic lesions. It is suggested that although this deformity is congenital, the manifestations are not present at birth because it is too early to recognize this deformity until the child becomes a little older and enters into some severe activities such as athletics. Then when an injury occurs, the pain becomes severe and the disability begins. It is believed that the talocalcaneal bridge is prone to cause more deformity than the calcaneo-navicular bar. The condition causes a certain amount of rigidity and movements at the midtarsal joint are considerably restricted. Pain is one of the most frequent symptoms when the injury takes place and this is the symptom in most instances that brings the patient into the office for treatment.

Muscle spasm, especially in the peroneus longus and in more severe cases, in the extensor digitorum longus, also develops at some stage of the disability. This spasm is brought on by activity and is relieved by rest. The degree of spasm is definitely related to the degree of use to which the foot is subjected. Peroneal muscle spasm can be confirmed by the use of anesthesia in the form of a peroneal nerve block at the point where the nerve crosses the posterior surface of the head of the fibula. Even though the spasm may be eliminated, the deformity and rigidity will remain and the pain is not completely relieved.

An injection into the sinus tarsi of the foot will relieve the residual pain. X-rays taken at the proper angles may not only reveal the intertarsal bridge but will also show secondary change in a region of the subtalar and talonavicular joints. Harris describes the technique for taking these X-rays as follows: "Medical talocalcaneal bridge can be demonstrated by projecting the x-ray beam from behind downward and forward through the joint between the sustentaculum tali and the neck of the talus. The patient stands on the film with the knee slightly flexed and the ankles slightly dorsiflexed. Three films should be exposed with the angle of projection of the X-ray beam at thirty, thirty-five and forty degrees to the surface on which the patient is standing. One of these projections will usually show the sustentacular joint space or reveal a bone bridge between the talus and calcaneus." This technique is illustrated in articles by Harris and Beath. The calcaneal navicular bar is best revealed by an oblique projection of the X-ray beam through the middle of the foot from a lateral to the medial side at an angle of forty-five degrees to the film on which the patient stands."

Dr. Harris suggests that since the amount of deformity and the degree of disablement by pain and muscle spasm are factors which vary greatly with patients who have peroneal spastic flatfoot, that in the milder problems conservative measures should be tried. He states that the best measure for both medial talocalcaneal bridge and calcaneal navicular bar is an accurately fitted Whitman plate. This plate will diminish the stress on the rigid tarsus and relieve pain and muscle spasm. However, when the degree of deformity and severity of pain cannot be relieved by conservative treatment, he believes that surgery is indicated. Surgery in these instances is designed to bring about complete fusion.

Joseph R. Cinzio presents the case histories of seven young adult patients with Freiberg's infraction of the second or third metatarsal heads, where he attempts to show a relationship between the Freiberg's infractions and arthritis involving the metatarsal-phalangeal joints of the foot. Enteric cortisone therapy was used with good results in all seven instances. Along with this therapy, Cinzio writes that metatarsal plates, felt padding, Thomas bars, balance inlays and physiotherapy are also efficacious in the treatment of this condition.

In summarizing his article on "The Role of the Os Tibiale Externum in Patho-Mechanical Disorders of the Foot," Murray Bromberg states: "The particular importance attaching to the presence of the os tibiale externum or accessory tarsal scaphoid lies, not in the presence of this accessory bone per se, but in the fact that it indicates an abnormal insertion of the tendon of the tibialis posterior, which may produce a weak foot, the tendon being entirely or mainly inserted into the navicular."

Frank A. Bersani and associates describe a massive tarsal synostosis appearing bilaterally in two successive generations of one family. In this description there was congenital bilateral fusion of the talus, the navicular, the cuboid, the middle and lateral cuneiforms, and the second, third, and fourth metatarsals. In this discussion, Bersani quotes that Shands and Wentz reviewed 850 roentgenograms of children's feet which demonstrated various deformities, and in this group six patients showed fusion of two or more tarsal bones. One of the patients showed bilateral fusion of all the tarsals except the first cuneiform. He also discusses several other authors who have described calcaneal-navicular and talonavicular coalition, particularly with reference to peroneal spasm.

Leonard H Lerner has gathered some interesting information on calcaneal apophysitis in the development of his article "Radiographic Evaluation of Calcaneal Apophysitis." He contends that "lack of adequate correlation between the X-ray findings and the clinical picture has been noted for some time by a number of investigators."

Over a period of years we have X-rayed hundreds of calcanei in order to verify the findings of calcaneal apophysitis and these findings have in no way differed from the findings of X-rays of calcanei for normal feet. When a child complains of a painful heel, the pain itself is most often localized in a small area at the posterior inferior medial aspect of the calcaneus and is not distributed over the entire epiphyseal cap area.

Lerner believes that it is localized in this area because of the trauma directed to this one specific spot. Furthermore, he does not believe that this trauma was induced by normal walking or running. In most instances the trauma was induced by jumping or by kicking the heels or by dragging the heels such as will happen quite often when boys are at play. The fact that this condition is rarely seen in girls is most significant because boys are far more active than girls in their athletic activities and play. Because of these clinical findings, we cannot agree that the condition we call calcaneal apophysitis is at all related to a vascular necrosis or aseptic necrosis. It is therefore not in the same category as Freiberg's disease or Kohler's disease; in fact, it should not be labeled a disease but simply classified as a traumatic experience to a growth segment of the bone structure.

Finally, we have never been confronted with a single instance of calcaneal apophysitis that has not responded to conservative therapy. This is not true with other areas of the body that are affected by aseptic necrosis.

Osgood-Schlatter's Disease

Osgood-Schlatter's disease, a synonym for osteochondrosis of the tibial tubercle, is usually found in young adolescents and is more prevalent in males than in females. Medial-lateral views of the upper section of the tibia will reveal a considerable amount of eburnation in the area of the tibial tubercle, and some spur-like formation and ossicle formations.

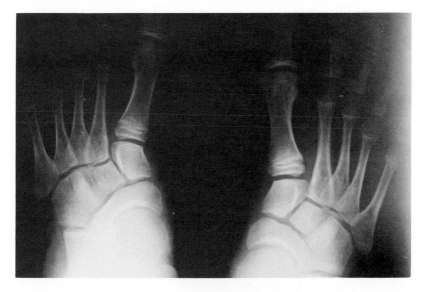

Fig. 97. X-ray of Sixteen Year Old Male—Spastic Flat Foot with Mid Tarsal
Bony Coalition.

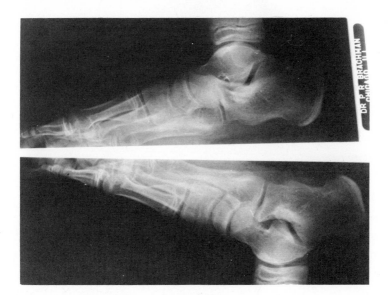

Fig. 98. Lateral X-ray Views of Same Patient.

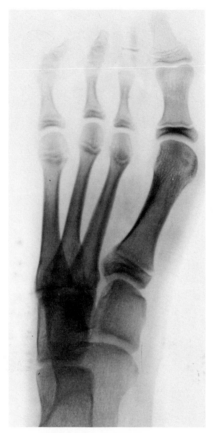

Fig. 99. X-ray of Young Male with Congenital Coalition of Calcaneus and
Talus.

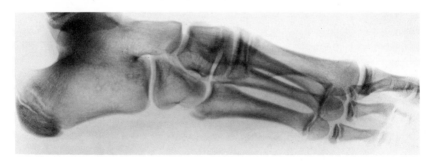

Fig. 100 Dorso-Plantar X-ray—Same Patient.

Bony Coalitions

In the foot a coalition is usually associated with one or two bones in the midtarsal area of the foot in which two or more bones are connected by a bridge of bone, cartilage, or fibrous tissue. The bony bridge is known as a synostosis; the ligamentous as syndesmosis; and the fibrous tissue as synchondrosis. While only the bony bridge can be demonstrated in X-rays taken at specific angles to show these coalitions, the diagnosis of a coalition in the midtarsal area or tarsal area of the foot is made clinically by peroneal spasms of the peroneal or extensor muscles with pain as the chief complaint.

Coalitions of this type are common and have been found in the foot dissections of fetuses from three months to five months of age. Because of this finding, these coalitions are thought to be hereditary. In most instances they cause no difficulty until the child becomes quite active, such as boys playing baseball. When the structure where the coalition exists becomes innured and the onset of symptoms appear, it becomes exceedingly difficult for the patient to move his foot normally when the symptom becomes symptomatic.

The normal range of eversion and inversion can be affected with the associated peroneal spasm, and the foot is generally held in a marked valgus position. Walking becomes painful and difficult and the patient requires a considerable amount of treatment in order to bring about some degree of correction. A Roberts plate of stainless steel fitted to the foot in order to keep it in a neutral position so that inversion and eversion will be eliminated is usually quite adequate after the initial treatment has eliminated the primary symptoms of pain.

18. METATARSUS VARUS

McCauley, in discussing "Recurrence in Congenital Metatarsus Varus," states: "The condition is usually considered to be quite docile, rarely or never recurring after treatment and even less frequently causing a significant therapeutic problem. It is our belief that there is a significant tendency toward recurrence of the deformity with eventual fixation of the foot in the adducted position. In addition, the presence of an unrecognized valgus deformity of the hind part of the foot is often unmasked during treatment. If not properly treated, a pronated foot results. Kite emphasized in the treatment of metatarsus varus that constant care must be exercised not to turn the heel out in a valgus position and that the foot must not be held in casts in the overcorrected position for too long a time or a flatfoot will be produced."

At the close of the article, under the section "Discussion," McCauley writes: "We believe this study has demonstrated that the treatment of congenital metatarsus varus presents problems that are not always appreciated. The apparently corrected foot can revert to a position of deformity if the corrective apparatus is discontinued too soon. It should be emphasized that the statistics are undoubtedly affected by certain variables in treatment. All feet were not treated in a uniform manner. It has been suggested by some that metatarsus varus hardly requires any therapy. To the contrary, it is our belief that definitive therapy is indicated and that it is often abandoned too quickly. Once the fully corrected position has been attained, the full eversion of the forepart of the foot is possible with no more force than would be necessary in the normal foot where a period of holding is indicated. The duration of this holding phase should range from three to six weeks depending upon the time necessary for original correction. This is particularly true in the younger patients whose deformity showed a somewhat greater tendency to recur. The second important finding in this study was the significant degree of valgus of the hind part of the foot in many feet treated for metatarsus varus. Although not all of the feet in which pronation developed were significantly deformed, some were. Eversion of the calcaneus must be avoided during the treatment phases as heel valgus and flatfoot are common sequelae of this disorder."

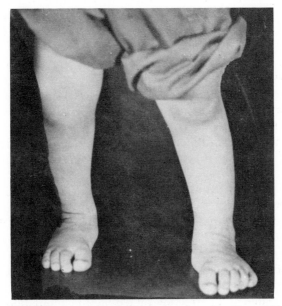

Fig. 101.   Accodative Pigeon-toeing—Six Year Old Male.

Accommodative Pigeon-toeing

We must disagree with this author and we contend that whenever children are examined for metatarsus varus or metatarsus adductus and an associated rear foot valgus is found in the same foot, we are dealing with a separate and different entity. This is the entity that we have labeled accommodative pigeon-toeing. Accommodative pigeon-toeing is not difficult to diagnose in children who are already standing and walking. In this condition, the forepart of the foot will be seen to turn in, but the rear foot will be seen to turn out into a valgus position. If the child is asked to run and can do so, the entire foot will be seen to assume the valgus attitude and the child will run as if the feet were pronated. Parents have often advised us that when their children who pigeon-toe most of the time become fatigued or tired, they walk with their feet in an abducted position similar to that of a marked pronation problem.

Since the primary factor here is rear foot valgus, we do not treat these children as we would the ordinary metatarsus adductus or metatarsus varus problems. In such cases we treat the rear foot problem and allow the forefoot to take its course which it will do if the rear foot is corrected. The diagnosis of this condition in infants who have not yet attempted weight bearing and walking is much more difficult. In such instances the examiner will have to determine, by means of examination of the range of motion of the various parts of the foot whether or not the condition is one of rear foot valgus or truly one of forefoot adduction. The treatment then will be designed to overcome the primary condition that exists.

At one point McCauley states: "It is customary to determine the rigidity of the deformity by its response to corrective force. When varus and valgus forces are applied to the metatarsal region with the calcaneus and talus fixed in neutral position, the range of motion of the midtarsal joint can be determined. If the front part of the foot cannot be brought into axial alignment with the heel, the deformity is said to be fixed. When the foot can be brought into axial alignment, the deformity is considered flexible and correction by parental manipulation is tried. The mild or attitudinal varus deformities, which can be completely or almost completely reversed by the examining physician, usually respond well to manipulation, if they are performed with intelligence and industry."

Our experience in examination of feet with these problems and in the treatment of attitudinal deformities does not correspond with the information as given by McCauley. In trying to determine the ranges of motion in dorsiflexion, plantarflexion, abduction, adduction, supination, and pronation, together with inversion and eversion, we find that some children develop a considerable degree of resistance to our efforts to induce these ranges of motion.

If we are not careful with our examinations and do not take a sufficient amount of time with each child, we will find ourselves listing deformities that actually do not exist. Some children become very tense during examination and resist all of our efforts to try to find a true relationship between ranges of motion at the various joints. Over a period of many years, we have asked parents to manipulate and stretch the feet of these young children where we considered the deformity to be mild and therefore possibly reversible. There have been very few instances where the results have been positive. In most of these children it has been our experience that it was necessary to apply more stringent corrective methods before correction could be achieved.

Oscar M. Scheimer discusses in a condensed fashion twelve case histories of infants between the ages of two months and eight months where he applied plaster of paris casts for treatment with results that were from good to excellent. It has long been our opinion that if the diagnosis is truly that of metatarsus varus and if the treatment is started at an early age, it is possible to bring about full correction within a period of one to three months with the use of our skates that we have described in other sections of this volume. The use of plaster of paris, especially in unilateral cases, does bring about some secondary changes in the development of the unaffected foot, as compared with that of the involved foot and leg. Furthermore, we also believe that the use of plaster of paris is related to the philosophy of immobilization, while the greatest benefits to be derived from the treatment with skate therapy is related to the philosophy of mobilization which brings about the correction under more normal physiological conditions.

19. PHYSICAL vs. CHRONOLOGICAL AGE

Weak Foot in Children

Because there are so many theories relating to basic foot difficulties in childhood, it is apparent that most of these theories are not based upon practical experience gained in the treatment of children's feet. It is the author's belief that too much attention has been directed towards physical age in children in relation to the development of the feet. Just because the textbook claims that the navicular begins to ossify at three years of age is no reason for us to assume that each and every child will develop as rapidly as every other child when the calendar proclaims them to be three years old. Instead, we must think in terms of physical age of these children rather than the chronological age.

In thinking of the physical age we may be confronted with the possibility of seeing a child who is six years old chronologically, but who is less than three years old physically from a foot developmental and foot functional standpoint. In other words, the child of six will show retardation of development of the navicular and cuneiforms. X-rays of children's feet will confirm this fact.

If it is true that children who do not bear their weight normally show marked deficiencies in the ossification time for normal children, then it must also be true that these children should not be expected to carry out the same active play program of the average child of that age. They should be restricted in their activities and their parents and teachers must be directed in the amount of restriction that the children should undergo. Longer periods of rest are necessary and it is almost needless to say that nutritional factors, especially vitamin and mineral therapy, should be considered.

Shoe Therapy for Children

Helfet, writing in Lancet, February 11, 1956, states that he has developed a corrective heel seat made from fiberglass which he has used on 500 children in the treatment of flat feet. He claims cures have been attained in all cases over an average time of two to two and one-half years of use. Helfet believes that the pigeon-toed gait is the child's attempt to correct the heel eversion, while the Charlie Chaplin gait is the child's attempt to walk the best that it knows how because it cannot overcome the eversion. He claims that he does not like to use arch supports and inlays because they are a supportive factor and also a weakening one on the musculature of the foot, and if prescribed for a child, constitute a life sentence. Helfet is also critical of the Thomas heel because he says it is not wholly effective in reforming the arch of the foot, and there must be a continuity of treatment if good results are to be expected. He contends that to be effective the shoes need constant repair and renewal.

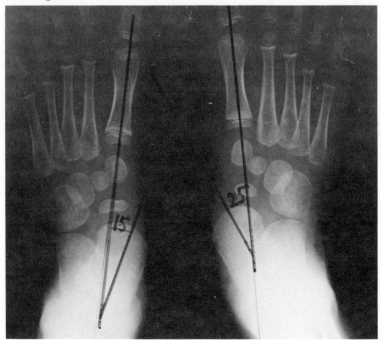

Fig. 102. Six Year Old Male with Mid-Tarsal Weakness and Retarded Navicular Development.

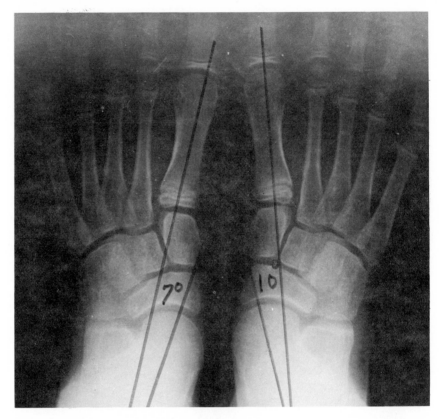

Fig. 103. Same Patient as Fig. 102 at Age Thirteen. Treated with Whitman Plates for Five Years.

If the diagnosis and treatment of foot problems in children were as simple as outlined by Helfet, it is possible that these problems could be corrected with Helfet's measures and with many other simple measures that are used from time to time by orthopedic men and podiatrists.

The attempt to correct these conditions by cupping the heel in a shoe is not new, and has been used for many years. There is no doubt that on some occasions and in some cases it is of considerable value, but it cannot be used universally as Helfet believes, as may be deducted from his discussion.

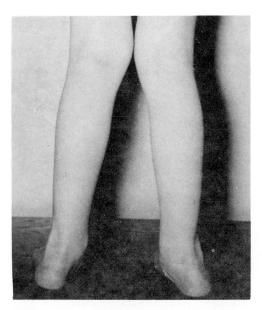

Fig. 104. Severe Weak Foot (Pes Plano Valgus) in Five Year Old Female with Genu Valgum.

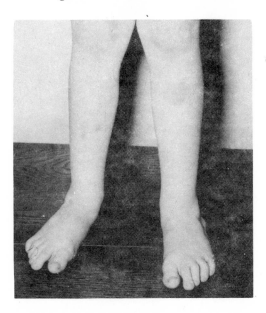

Fig. 105. Same Patient—Front View.

Plaster Casting for Weak Foot

Darby advocates casting as a new approach for the correction of congenital pronation in infants. Darby has observed some good results casting infants for this problem, as have many others over the years. It is our opinion, however, as has been expressed in other pages of this text and others we have developed, that positive diagnostic procedures revealing the true etiology of the factors producing pronation make it unnecessary to apply casts to the foot at any stage.

We believe that whenever plaster of paris is used on the foot or for any other part of the body for the correction of a condition, we are not dealing with an inocuous type of therapy. Whenever a part of the body is encased in plaster of paris, that part becomes immobilized and immobility will always produce some definite loss in the function and metabolism and a further loss in circulatory efficiency. Because motion is completely inhibited the restriction of joint movement always endangers the synovia within the joint. It has been reported experimentally that keeping a joint immobile for a minimum of six days will produce destructive forces that to some degree can never be reversed.

There is also the problem of immobilizing one foot while the other requires no attention; if this continues for a period of weeks or months, the foot requiring no attention and the leg above it will certainly show signs of disuse atrophy which remain for the rest of the patient's lifetime. This can be observed in patients who have had this type of therapy for unilateral clubfoot during infancy and are now adults.

20. CEREBRAL PALSY IN INFANTS AND CHILDREN

An Introduction to the Problem of Cerebral Palsy

Cerebral palsy may be defined as a disease seen at birth or in early infancy and is characterized by a disturbance of voluntary motor function. The essential pathology is a destruction or congenital absence of neurons in the cerebellum or cerebrum. Cerebral palsy is to be suspected if the newborn infant does not breathe well, fails to nurse, remains bluish in color, has convulsions, or shows marked weakness or tightness of the muscles. The most common cause of the destruction of the brain cells is thought to be hemorrhage into the brain prior to or immediately following birth. Anoxia of the brain in utero is also considered to be responsible for much of the brain damage.

In many instances nothing unusual is noticed about the child at birth until it becomes obvious that the child cannot hold its head, sit up, stand, or walk in the same time sequence as that carried out by normal children. He is unable to relax his muscles normally, and his movements are jerking, labored and inaccurately executed. The area of the brain damage in spasticity lies near the motor area and sufficient destruction may occur to produce varying degrees of mental retardation. However, retardation can also be present due to the physical handicap, as a result of which the child finds it difficult to express himself.

Numerically the problem of cerebral palsy is significant for it is estimated that there are more than 400,000 in the United States. Although the subject of cerebral palsy has been neglected in our medical literature, we are beginning to lift the curtain of confusion that has hidden this condition for many years.

173

Classification

Most authorities now agree that cerebral palsy may be classified according to the anatomic site of the brain lesion, the clinical picture, the impairment of the extremities, the degree of tonicity, the severity of the involvement and the etiology.

The site of the brain involved covers three general categories:

1. Pyramidal tract problems are most often true spastics and the clinical syndromes are thought to be due to the removal of the inhibitory effects of the pyramidal tracts.
2. Extrapyramidal tract problems are primarily associated with athetosis, choreas, tremors, ballismus, dystonias, and rigidities.
3. Cerebellum problems are most often associated with ataxics and atonias.

The most accepted clinical classification divides all cerebral palsy patients into five primary groups: spastics, athetoids, tremors, ataxics and rigidities.

1. *Spastic Type.* In this type the pathology to the brain affects the muscle directly and the "stretch reflex" is a special characteristic which distinguishes this type. When a normal muscle contracts its antagonist must relax, allowing the muscle tone to become lowered enough to allow the desired motion to be carried out. This phenomenon is known as Sherrington's Law of Reciprocal Innervation. In contrast, the spastic muscle is hyper-irritable and reacts to any stimulus by contracting not only the agonist, but the antagonist as well.

Another diagnostic feature of the spastic is the "cerebral zero" or $0°$ C. muscle. These muscles have no power to carry out function and they are not generally found in the other forms of cerebral palsy. To test for such a muscle the muscle should be put into the contracted position by the operator and if the patient is unable to hold it in that position voluntarily it must be recorded as $0°$ C.

The equinus limp is another frequent finding. This finding is not due to the weakness of the dorsiflexors but to the simultaneous contraction of the more powerful plantarflexors. This is particularly true of the hemiplegic spastic who can usually walk, but the affected leg will drag and is not too useful.

The scissors gait or cross-legged progression gait is associated most often with the paraplegic and quadriplegic types. This gait is characterized by a disabling adduction of the hips due to the greater strength of the adductor groups of muscles. When this persists other characteristic deformities develop as time goes on. The hips may become flexed, adducted and internally rotated. The knees are flexed and the feet assume an equinus or equinovarus position.

2. *Athetoid Type*. Athetosis has been described as "a condition in muscles which brings about contractions without voluntary direction, and without voluntary control." The athetosis involves the involuntary motions only and the voluntary motions are not affected. The athetoid who makes no effort to stop these involuntary motions is known as a nontension athetoid while the athetoid who voluntarily tenses to stop these involuntary motions is called a tension athetoid.

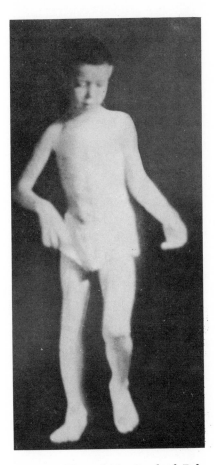

Fig. 106. Hemiplegic Cerebral Palsy
—Age Nine—Right Side Involved.

In the athetoid the damage in the brain is to the basal ganglia which control the joints of the body. The ganglia act as a filter and sort out desired motions. When these are damaged the sorting function is interfered with and all impulses pass through causing involuntary motion in all parts of the body. The ability to control motion at will is lost. Feeble-mindedness, if found, has no direct relationship to the athetoid condition.

Generally speaking the athetoid must be slowed down, while the spastic is a slow-moving child and must be speeded up.

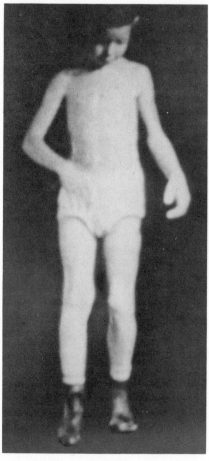

Fig. 107. Hemiplegic Cerebral with Surgical Shoes and Inlays Accommodating Shortage on Left.

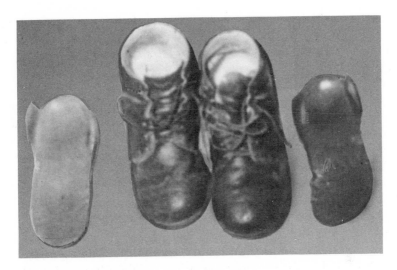

Fig. 108. Shoes and Inlays for Patient Fig. 106.

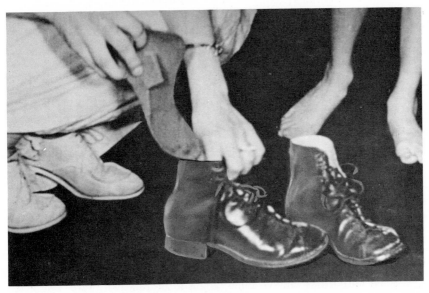

Fig. 109. Second View of Shoes and Inlays for Patient Fig. 106.

3. *Tremor Type*. This is a type related to the athetoid in which the motion not only returns to the neutral stage but goes beyond, into overflexion and overextension. Intentional tremors occur during a voluntary attempt to move at will. Unintentional tremors are more or less constant and occur at all times.

4. *Ataxic Type*. Ataxia is caused by damage to the cerebellum—the brain center controlling coordination of movements. The kinesthetic sense, which is the ability to know the position of joints in relation to other parts of the body, is lost. Control of direction and force of motion is difficult once voluntary action is begun. These patients must be treated by training other motor centers to take over the work of the impaired area.

5. *Rigid Type*. This type is characterized by a stiffness in the muscles of the arms and legs with no involuntary motions or stretch reflex present. Muscles respond slowly and with difficulty when a stimulus is applied. Rigidity appears to be caused by a diffuse lesion of the brain and occurs often after a convulsive seizure. The muscles may be rigid in the flexed and extended positions.

Cerebral palsy may be further classified on the basis of the topographical distribution of the involvement. The incidence of the impairment of the extremities has been listed as follows for the most commonly used terms:

1. Quadriplegia—all four extremities—60%
2. Hemiplegia—arm and leg on one side—20%
3. Monoplegia—single extremity involved—10%
4. Paraplegia—both legs involved—10%

It is thought that patients with quadriplegia who have most of the involvement in the legs are usually spastics and those with the arms primarily involved are athetoids.

The problem in hemiplegics affects one half of the body. While it is presumed that all hemiplegics are spastics, pure hemiplegic athetoids have been reported. Some hemiplegics present an atrophy of the affected arm and leg resulting in a shortage of one or both. These cannot be explained on a disuse basis and must be presumed to be congenital in origin. There may also be a sensory involvement on the affected side. Proprioception, two-point discrimination and form perception may be affected.

Some authorities believe monoplegia to be relatively rare, but when it does occur it is believed to be spastic in nature.

Paraplegics are thought to be of the spastic variety in almost all instances.

The change in muscle tone is also one of the characteristic findings in the cerebral palsy patient. Physiologically, the state of the muscle can be classified as:

1. Having normal tone—isotonic
2. Having increased tone—hypertonic
3. Having decreased tone—hypotonic or atonic.

All types of cerebral palsy patients may present these varied muscle tones to a more or less marked degree and that must be taken into consideration when making the diagnosis, prognosis, and deciding on the treatment.

We have already stated that cerebral palsy patients can also be classified according to the degree of involvement present. This classification can fall into the three grades of mild, moderate and severe and its importance is most apparent to those who treat such patients clinically. The significance of this classification will become apparent in this thesis.

The final classification that can be of considerable value to the total analysis of the subject is the classification according to etiology. A division of this classification into prenatal, natal and postnatal factors must be apparent.

A. Prenatal—may be due to genetic defects or to injuries acquired in utero.
   1. Hereditary—genetically transmitted
      a. Static—symptoms are present at birth and do not progress. Examples are, familial tremors, hereditary athetosis and familial spastic paraplegia.
      b. Progressive—symptoms may or may not be present at birth but may appear in later years. These are progressive and generally fatal—Tay-Sachs disease, demyelinating disease and tuberous sclerosis.
   2 Acquired in Utero—
      a. Prenatal infection
      b. Prenatal anoxia
      c. Prenatal cerebral hemorrhage
      d. Rh factor
      e. Metabolic disturbance
      f. Gonadal irradiation.

B. Natal factors—Those factors operating during the period of delivery of the child.
  1. Anoxia
  2. Cerebral hemorrhage and contusions
C. Postnatal factors—Factors operating after birth.
  1. Trauma
  2. Infections of the Central Nervous System
  3. Toxic causes including chemical poisoning
  4. Vascular accidents
  5. Anoxia
  6. Neoplastiç or late developmental defects

The General Foot Problem

All cerebral palsy children require constant proper pediatric care and they all respond in some measure to the various methods employed by physical medicine. While foot problems are only a part of the total difficulties that must be dealt with in the care of such children, these problems present a challenge to the medical team and it is in this category that the podiatrist can be a distinct asset to that team endeavor.

When we consider cerebral palsy children from the podiatry point of view we can divide all patients into three primary categories: those who have so little functional possibilities that they may never be able to bear their own body weight in the upright position; those who will walk with some degree of marked handicap at some time or other before puberty, and those who can walk with a mild degree of handicap at an early age.

It is logical to assume that we cannot be of much help to the first group, most of whom may become institutionalized sooner or later. The other two groups can use our services to advantage. In these two groups we must direct our attention to the task of preventing deformity where there is any indication that it may develop, overcoming deformity where it already exists, and adding to the general comfort and well-being of the patient by means of general prophylactic care of the feet.

Working with cerebral palsy children requires many years of attention and supervision of each individual case. Only then can we be assured that these children will be able to stand and walk well enough to take their places in our community as useful citizens. Such a program can be carried out best by a complete team effort of medical men and all affiliated medical services.

Skate Therapy

It has been twenty years since the author treated his first very young cerebral palsy patient for what was essentially a problem affecting the gait of the child. For several years we had been working with a mechanical device attached to surgical shoes which produced very favorable results in children with talipes equinovarus, talipes equino-varus, talipes equinovalgus, talipes varus and calcaneovalgus. As a result of this work we saw many young patients with problems other than those listed and it was inevitable that we should see some cerebral palsy children among them.

Within a period of five years after the first patient, we saw more than twenty-five patients with a variety of problems associated with cerebral palsy, and as the result of some trial and error therapy we arrived at some basic findings about the treatment that we could use with some success.

In 1949 we gave a short talk on the subject of "skate" therapy. In that talk we stated the following: "The cerebral palsy problem came to us slowly at first, but in the past few years, with the entire country more and more aware of this childhood malady, we are compelled to turn our attention to cerebrals of all types. The problems of aiding the cerebral child to walk is to some extent our problem. There was a time when the authorities on cerebral palsy paid little attention to the walking problem but it is realized today that the cerebral child who can walk best will improve more rapidly in all other aspects also."

"With these patients the skates are employed as a device to encourage a physiologically correct neuromuscular training program. Since the normal pathways from the brain to the periphery are destroyed or impaired, a fairly good substitute pathway can be set up with constant usage of the skates and other encouragement. The appliances prevent the patient from performing any exaggerated movements and control the gait to a fairly normal range of movement.

"The use of the skates on cerebrals has been most gratifying because of the results which have been obtained in a number of patients. We have applied these skates to patients from three to five years of age who have never been able to stand alone or take a step unaided and within six months to one year these children were able to stand unaided and take steps unaided. This aspect of the work has been most encouraging and we hope that the use of the skates will become more widespread than ever in the care of cerebral palsy patients."

The term "skates" in this thesis requires some explanation and description. Originally these devices were called the Brachman Talipes Splints or Reciprocal Ambulatory Skid Plates. They consisted of two sliding metal bars which were sandwiched between two aluminum plates attached firmly to each shoe. The device was so constructed that the patient was allowed to use his feet only in a pre-determined range of motion, usually an overcorrected range, as prescribed by the doctor.

The skates were most efficient when they were attached to a surgical type shoe because such shoes are constructed well enough to stand up under the wear and tear they receive. Furthermore, these shoes have open lacings to the end of the toes and it is not too difficult to place a contorted foot into the shoe. There were five basic types of skates designed to care for five specific foot and leg patterns associated with unilateral and bilateral problems. These five factors, multiplied by the many individual factors that must be included with each prescription, made it necessary from the very start to construct each pair on an individual basis.

Thus, each pair of skates were made and attached to each shoe by hand as ordered by the doctor, and they were so designed that they could not be changed unless they were returned to the laboratory under the order of the doctor. When we first designed these skates we found that if the parents of these patients were amateur mechanics they could reset the angle of correction at their own discretion and we were compelled to freeze the amount of correction in self-defense.

In using the skates the patient was taught how to move them. The doctor instructed the parents in the best technique designed to teach the child. The amount of activity indulged in by the patient was prescribed by the doctor, because it was obviously necessary to limit the activity to a few minutes in each hour if the structures were very weak and not accustomed to bearing weight. This time element was increased gradually from week to week.

Basically the skates allow the patient to perform most of the movements associated with locomotion, thus using the principles of mechanics that are physiologically correct. More specifically, the skates may be said to carry out the following physiological principles:

1. In normal walking we use one foot at a time and the young child obtains no more than eight to ten square inches of base support from each foot. When using the skates both feet are always in contact with the floor and this base area of support includes the entire parallelogram of not less than 100 square inches. This factor alone induces the patient

to balance himself once he finds it easier to do so and loses his fear of falling.

2. All undesirable movements are restricted and new and more desirable habit patterns affecting the neuromuscular pathways are developed. By so doing we may be blocking off the early patterns established by the brain pathology present and we may be using some of the more normal associated pathways for our locomotion. While this is now just conjecture, it may be established by future investigation. The fact that these changes occur is of major interest to us at the present time. Because these skates are worn day and night from the very start, the training program is uninterrupted and the new pattern has an excellent chance to become established on a more or less permanent basis. Of course, all of these factors also depend on the cooperation offered by the parents of the children we are treating.

3. All tightened and contracted structures are stretched with every movement that is made while the skates are worn.

An Approach to Treatment

To facilitate this broad problem of the approach to the foot care of the cerebral palsy child and young adult, we will describe what can best be done for these patients on the basis of the severity of the involvement. Earlier in this chapter we have classified these patients into three groups: mild, moderate and severe.

Since the mild group includes all those patients who are able to walk, use their arms and speak fairly well, our contact with them, clinically or as private patients, is rather limited. Their foot problems and gait problems appear to be no greater than those of our average citizens and it is only when they become injudicious in their activities that they require attention.

In most instances their problems are associated with early fatigue, limitation of range of motion and some loss of proprioceptive and kinesthetic sense. A close neurological and muscular examination together with a good case history will aid considerably in making the diagnosis. In treating such patients it must be remembered that we cannot replace what was never there to begin with, just as in the more severe types. Our attention, therefore, must be directed toward palliative treatment plus giving them some mechanical advantages through the use of mechanical therapy.

In the severe type, where there is total involvement and the patient is either bedridden or confined to a wheel chair and where the prognosis is very poor, the amount of good that we can do is negligible. However, it is very difficult to make a totally morbid prognosis for the very young child because there are so many factors that may change the situation after a few years' time. During the four years that we were associated with the Mercy Clinic we saw several children make some progress who appeared almost hopeless in infancy and we have also seen other children deteriorate as they became older.

Thus, as podiatrists, our basic approach to all infants and very young cerebrals must be hopeful. Where there are signs of impending foot and leg deformity we must try to prevent them and where they already exist when we first see these children we must correct them so that as the child gets older and the time comes for the first phase of locomotion to be developed, there will be no major deformity as a factor to be considered.

It is in the third, or moderate group, that we can do our very best work. This is the group where the involvement is always severe enough to handicap the patient in locomotion. Out of an active patient list of about 250 attending the clinic more than ninety were directed to our care for special foot and gait problems. Of these patients forty-one wore reciprocal skates, from one to three years. The remaining forty-nine patients received mechanical aids that ranged from shoe therapy to balance inlays, shortage devices and metal therapy.

Because the care and treatment of a cerebral palsy child require the services of a medical team, it is essential that the podiatrist who desires to take his place on this team sit in on a sufficient number of examinations and conferences so that he will understand and appreciate every phase of the problem. At the Mercy Clinic we had access to all of the examinations and conferences in progress together with the medical charts pertaining to each patient. Thus we were fully aware of the total problem of each patient. In most instances, that also included the family problems and the psychological problems which are almost always present.

We have found that the most important of all clinical conferences we attended were in conjunction with the examinations conducted by the physiatrists. Their basic approach to the problems of rehabilitation is so closely allied to our own work that we can work in harmony every step of the way. We made an effort to be present at the physical examination of each new patient by the physiatrist. At the completion of the examination we were usually invited to take over and re-examine the patient from a podiatric point of view. In each instance that examination included reflexes, range of motion, muscular function and an evaluation of basic walking patterns existing or likely to become activated. At this point we conferred with the physiatrist on the best therapeutic approach for locomotion or any other foot problem present.

It must be apparent by now that our approach to these various problems must have become somewhat standardized over a period of four years and to some extent that was quite true. The cerebral palsy patient is no different in that respect than any other patient. Certain problems fall into categories almost automatically with only the degree of severity serving as the greatest variant. Here again we would do best to follow a classification in our discussion and the topographical pattern plus the clinical symptoms will become our best guide.

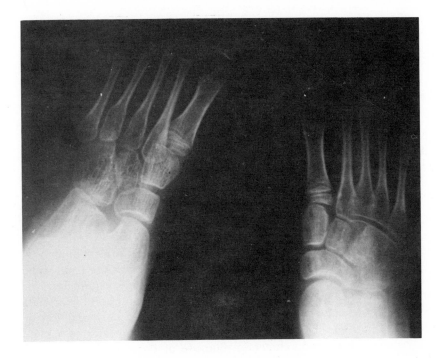

Fig. 110. Dorso-Plantar X-ray View of Left Hemiplegic Cerebral Palsy—Right Normal.

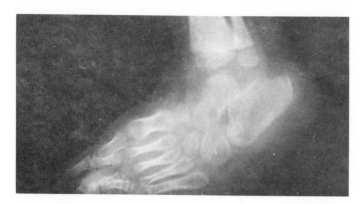

Fig. 111. Medial Lateral X-ray View of Left Hemiplegic Cerebral Palsy.

Spastic Hemiplegic

The spastic hemiplegics are an easily distinguishable group even at a very early age. The mechanics of one entire side of the body are affected and the child fails to use the affected hand but prefers to use the hand on the unaffected side. At six months the affected foot may show signs of an impending talipes equinovarus position. Furthermore, all reflexes are exaggerated on the affected side and the encephalogram will verify the damage done to only half of the affected brain area.

If these children were not treated and left to their own devices as they were years ago, they would grow up with very little or limited use of the extremities on the affected side. In most instances the hand would be useless and the foot would assume a marked talipes equinovarus position ending up in a complete deformity with fixation of all the articular structures. In many instances there is an associated knee and hip deformity which may be present very early or show up later as a factor associated with improper function. Because of the marked malfunction that exists there is always an associated shortage syndrome of the limb on the affected side. All of these factors require consideration in a planned course of treatment.

Quadriplegic

Of all the cerebral palsy patients the spastic quadriplegics probably make up the largest group. We have already stated that the very severe cases are not within the scope of the podiatrist's help once it has been established that the patient is nonambulatory. The more moderate cases can use our services with considerable benefit as long as they live.

The quadriplegic spastic has no single peculiarity of gait. He may begin to show signs of ambulation at an early age and often learns how to walk before two to three years of age, and again he may not take his first steps until the seventh year or later. The ability of this patient to walk is always dependent upon his ability to control his head and trunk muscles first. It is axiomatic that no spastic can walk before he learns to control his upper extremity.

When that control has been achieved, often after a great deal of effort on the part of the medical team and the family, then the patient is ready to walk, or at least make an effort to learn. What are the problems associated with the extremities of the spastic quadriplegic that may require attention? First and foremost there is always the inequality of the muscles due to the innervational overload affecting some of the muscles while others may actually register zero. The stretch reflex is always present with the true cerebral spastic. Whereas in a normal muscle a response to a stimulus will bring with it a contraction of the stimulated muscle and a relaxation of the antagonist, the spastic muscle will produce a contraction of both the agonist and the antagonist resulting in a sort of stalemate of activity. In other words, the antagonist opposes the normal action of the agonist.

With this lack of coordination going on between certain muscles and muscle groups one can readily visualize how difficult it becomes to initiate normal movement. Breaking up this stretch reflex pattern is a very difficult and tedious procedure and some muscles never respond favorably to any form of therapy used as a routine procedure. Of all therapies the one universally used at the present time includes all forms of massage and manipulation, often preceded by warm tub soaks or other forms of heat to induce some relaxation of the soft structures.

Dr. Karel Bobath and his wife, members of a British medical team, have had some success with a form of restraint therapy followed by rehabilitation exercises. By inhibiting the unorthodox movements through restraint they weaken the muscles to the point where they cannot resist passive normal motions. By this method they hope to give the patients an opportunity to become acquainted with the normal movements until they can carry them out of their own accord. Dr. Bobath's method of therapy is being used at a few clinic centers in the United States and the results are now being watched with a great deal of interest. The reports emanating from these centers are optimistic but not enough information has been gathered as yet to make any positive statements concerning the merit of this method of treatment.

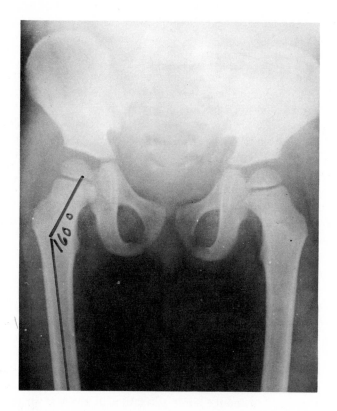

Fig. 112. Pelvic X-ray of Twelve Year Old Cerebral Palsy Patient with Partial Weight Bearing. Normal Structural Angle Between Neck and Shaft of Femur is 130 Degrees.

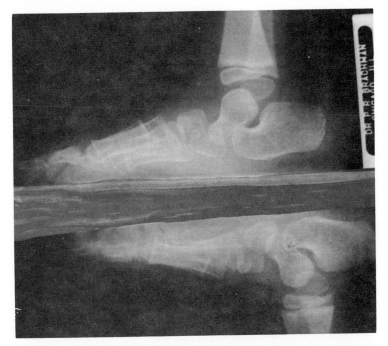

Fig. 113. X-ray View of Feet for Patient Fig. 112—Note Plantar Tali.

The spastic patient presents a large variety of foot problems and associated knee and hip problems from early infancy. There may be a unilateral or a bilateral talipes equinovarus, talipes equinovalgus, talipes varus, talipes valgus, calcaneovalgus, or talipes calcaneus. There may also be a talipes varus problem of one foot and a talipes valgus problem of the opposite foot. In other words, any possible combination of deformity problems may exist in the same patient. Associated with such foot problems we may also find hyperflexion or hyperextension of one or both knees, coxa vara or coxa valga of one or both hips, and a marked inward or outward rotation deformity of one or both limbs. It is also possible for one limb to be outward rotated with the opposite limb having a severe inward rotation problem.

As a general rule the digits of the toes are almost always involved with the primary problem associated with the hallux. The first digit usually shows the effects of a weakened extensor digitorum longus and

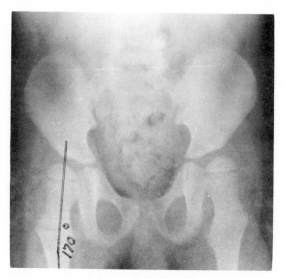

Fig. 114. Pelvic X-ray of Eleven Year Cerebral Palsy—Non Ambulatory
Patient. Angle of Neck and Shaft of Fermur, due to Lack of Weight
Bearing.

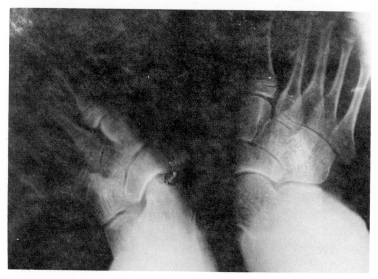

Fig. 115. Severe Malformation of Bony Foot Structures Resulting from Lack
of Functional Weight Bearing—Same as Fig. 114.

a spastic flexor hallucis longus. With all of these problems so often affecting the spastic patient it is little wonder that they never develop normal articulations as they grow older. Neither do they ever achieve normal balance and a coordinate walking pattern.

Finally, as these patients grow older, those who do get around develop pressure areas that need constant attention by the podiatrist in order to give the utmost comfort and stability. With all of the neurological problems already attendant with their spasticity, any other painful areas that are present on their feet may become an insurmountable factor in their effort to remain ambulatory. These patients require all of the patience and skills at our command to give them palliative relief by means of our surgical skills, mechanical aids and shoe therapy.

Athetoids

The term "athetoid" is applied to a third group of cerebral palsy patients. The numbers in this group may be equal to those listed as spastics, but in general, the total involvements are not as severe.

As we have stated previously, these patients are affected primarily by involuntary, uncontrollable and inco-ordinate movements. These movements may take on any bizarre pattern and may be slow or rapid, sudden or jerky in character. Most of these patients learn how to walk despite this handicap but their problems multiply with increased activity. The mild athetoid gets along fairly well with all activities but the more severe athetoid experiences difficulty with all factors relating to foot care, from just lacing and tying his shoes to simple prophylactic care.

Many athetoids experience similar problems with maintaining balance that affect the cerebral palsy group in general and moderate to severe foot and leg deformities develop with time as malstructure follows malfunction. Talipes problems, knee problems, hip rotational problems and the lesser problems generally seen by the podiatrist can all be present and must be properly diagnosed and treated.

Skate therapy has been used with very good results in the treatment of young athetoid patients and we have extended the use of skate therapy for the care of young adult athetoid patients with striking results. In most instances even the older athetoid patients do not present true deformities or contractures. Theirs is primarily a positional deformity and the skates, with their ability to restrain undesirable movements and direct the activity into new and more desirable neuromuscular patterns, apparently overcome this problem to a considerable degree. As far as our knowledge goes, no other therapy has been able to accomplish so much in so short a time for these patients and in most instances the adult problem was thought to be entirely hopeless.

Ataxics

The fourth classification we shall consider are the ataxics. The pure ataxic patient is not seen often. As has been stated previously, the disturbance of balance and equilibrium are the outstanding symptoms found in this group. Their kinesthetic sense is greatly impaired. Other than that they have few of the other symptoms found in most cerebral palsy patients.

The ataxic patient has an unsteady gait and falls frequently if he is not very careful. His main problem is to learn how to control his balance and be careful of the terrain over which he is walking. We have not had the opportunity to use any other special appliances on these patients other than balance inlays and they have been of some value.

Investigations Conducted and Planned

In February of 1955 we requested permission from the medical and clinical directors of the Mercy Hospital Rehabilitation Center to make a slow motion picture study of normal gaits and pathological gaits in young children, using the children attending our clinics as the subject material for this study. Approval was granted and we completed this pilot study in May of 1955.

The subjects were a normal five-year-old girl, a thirty-month-old quadriplegic spastic girl, a three-year-old athetoid girl, a nine-year-old hemiplegic boy and a seven-year-old ataxic boy. All of the cerebral palsy children could walk by themselves with varying degrees of stability and all were of sufficient intelligence to carry out most of the orders that were directed to them.

Since we required special slow motion camera equipment for this study, we were fortunate in receiving such assistance from the Illinois Institute of Technology. They supplied a technician and a Fastex camera, capable of taking moving pictures at any speed up to seven thousand frames a second. Our study was made at a speed of three hundred frames a second which was twenty times the speed of normal motion. The picture produced was slowed down to one-twentieth of the normal rate of motion.

This study gave us more than 800 feet of film depicting facts about normal and pathological gait that had not been observed before by any of the men in the medical specialties or allied medical fields, but the pilot effort that we were able to execute was only proof of the fact that a great deal more of this same investigation must be continued. Some of the facts learned by this study appear in the text in this chapter.

For many centuries medicine and its allied professions have been proud of the factual evidence they have been able to produce in all branches of practice. While the organized care of the cerebral palsy patient has a history of less than 45 years, there are very few facts that can be presented in the treatment of these patients where one could say with certainty "this method, if used according to all details listed, will bring results in thirty or forty or fifty per cent of the cases." Almost all the work that has been done is described with the appendage of "we think this is so" or "we believe this to be true." In other words the entire program has been lacking in factual proof.

We hope that insofar as the foot and gait problems are concerned, we have been able to bring some substantial evidence to bear concerning certain facts relating to treatment. When we first attended the clinics we became aware that all examinations of the lower extremity were made with the child in the sitting or in the prone position, regardless of the fact that the child could or could not bear some weight with or without help. Because the feet are greatly responsible for a share of the proprioceptive sense and balance mechanism of the body, and also because the action of the muscles on weight bearing are greatly altered in their actions as observed in the rest position, it is imperative that the examinations be carried out in both positions wherever feasible.

Weight bearing sets up normal reflex arcs that are never found in the rest position and these reflexes also are of great importance in the understanding of the mechanism of locomotion. It is our belief that the most important of these is the Babinski reflex. While we know of it only as a diagnostic sign it is far more than that. The Babinski response can be obtained by activating the motor reflex arc at any point on the plantar or dorsal area of the foot. Because of the fact that the cerebral patient is hypersensitive and has a great overflow of motor response going to some muscles, weight bearing alone may produce extrasensory stimulation that will be entirely different from the rest picture. By the

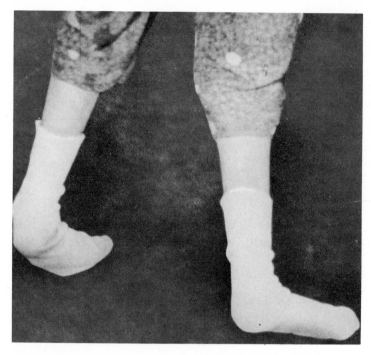

Fig. 116. Quadriplegic Cerebral Female—Age Sixteen—Right Foot Severe
    Talipes Equino Valgus—Left Foot Talipes Equino Varus. Patient
    Cannot Walk Unaided.

same token it is also possible, by mechanical means, to inhibit some of
these extrasensory factors and to stimulate others that may be more
normal in scope.

In testing both spastic and athetoid children to determine whether
we could elicit a certain reflex response at will by digital pressure, we
applied pressure to the talonavicular articulation wherever we met with
a peroneal spasm that held the foot in the range of marked abduction.
This was the type of abduction that was associated with a stretch reflex
and where the foot could be brought back to a normal alignment only
after severe force was applied. In practically every instance, pressure
at the talonavicular articulation set up a reflex response that released
the spasm and allowed us to bring the foot into normal alignment with
very little or no effort.

In applying this finding practically, we placed a high fulcrum into the shoes of these patients under the talonavicular articulation and achieved similar results on weight bearing. Then we designed balance inlays for these children carrying out the same principle with equally good results. In other words, the same reflex mechanism that produced the Babinski phenomenon was also used as a mechanical advantage in normal weight bearing and walking.

While the investigation and work that we have done to establish the validity of our hypothesis that reflexes in the feet are not just there to give us a diagnostic factor has been very limited, we are continuing this line of investigation with the addition of another hypothesis. It is our belief that all cerebral palsy children, and possibly other children with associated neurological disturbances, who cannot perform the initial functions of locomotion should receive the benefit of pressure therapy directed to the soles of the feet so as to activate or initiate the reflex response that is associated with direct weight bearing.

We hope to have more information to offer on this subject at a later date, but at the present time it does offer many interesting avenues for investigation for those who wish to avail themselves of what such an hypothesis may reveal.

We would like to devote some space to another problem that has been of interest to us and one to which we have devoted a considerable amount of time and thought during the past few years. We refer to the definite relationship that exists between the development of all factors of active walking in the normal infant and child to that of the cerebral palsy child. Our observations and study have lead us to the conclusion that all normal children conform to the following pattern in learning how to walk:

1. Between four and seven months of age most children begin to develop reciprocal motion in both legs. This function becomes so well coordinated that if most children of seven months of age are held up in the erect position their little legs will move reciprocally as if they are ready to take off and walk without any effort.

2. From the seventh through the 12th month, most children develop the balance phase so essential for weight-bearing and locomotion. They are able to raise themselves from the floor and by holding on they can achieve a good degree of balance.

3. From the twelfth to the twentieth month most children learn to walk without any further aid as follows:

a. The first steps are hesitating and awkward with the child falling often.

b. The stance is wide with the feet and legs widespread for greater stability.

c. The knees are flexed.

d. Most of the weight thrust is on the forefoot.

4. As the child continues to gain more confidence, the widespread stance disappears, the child falls less often, the knees no longer flex and the weight thrust comes down on the heel with the initiation of each step.

Now let us analyze the gait of the cerebral palsy child from the very beginning.

1. He may take from one to seven years or more to learn reciprocal leg motion.

2. He may require one to five years in addition before he gains sufficient balance to enable him to stand alone.

3. When some degree of walking actually becomes an accomplished fact, his gait will always have the following characteristics to some degree unless some drastic steps are taken to bring about desirable changes:

a. His steps will remain hesitating and awkward and he will be subject to frequent falls.

b. His stance will be widespread for greater stability.

c. His knees will remain flexed in most instances.

d. Most of the weight thrust will be on the forefoot and he will remain a toe-heel walker.

e. Partial ankylosis of the hip joints may bring about further complications in the gait problem.

It now becomes obvious how the cerebral pattern follows that of the normal child in everything except timing up to a certain point. That point is reached when the normal child is ready to iron out the rough spots in his gait from the 18th through the 24th month. The cerebral never irons out these rough spots and to a greater degree keeps them for a lifetime.

What can we as podiatrists do to help the cerebral iron out some of these rough spots in his attempt to walk more normally? We require more information about the development of the walking processes of the normal child. Such a study should be undertaken on an independent basis by a number of organizations and institutions but all should co-ordinate their efforts so that there will not be too much duplication of effort.

Because of the fact that skate therapy has resulted in the creation of a more normal pattern of walking by virtue of its restraining action, the creation of new reflex habit patterns approaching the normal, and its ability to bring the heel down from its elevated position, we should urge all those interested in this problem to include this therapy wherever it is indicated. Finally, we can use all of the modalities of physical therapy at our disposal to aid in the rehabilitation process so essential to the successful treatment of the cerebral palsy patient.

We have been deliberate in refraining from a discussion of surgery for the prevention or the correction of deformities in the cerebral palsy patient because most evidence now points to the fact that surgery has only a minor place in this entire program. We would prefer, therefore, to let others offer a critical analysis of its value or lack of value.

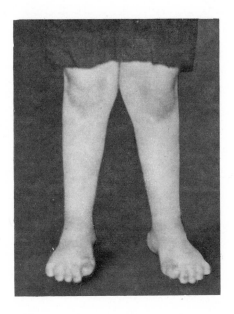

Fig. 117. Milder Cerebral Palsy Quadriplegic—Note Dorsiflexion of Great Toes.

Chart Relating to "Skate" Therapy for Twenty-One Cases Selected from Clinic Files

Patient Number	Age	Sex	Length of Time Skates Were Used—in Months	Improvement of Balance or Walking	Improvement of Limb Rotation	Improvement of Equinus Position	Diagnosis—Type of Cerebral Palsy
1	4.6 mo.	M	9	Good	Good	Excellent	Spastic Quad.
2	4	F	12	Good	Excellent	Excellent	Spastic Quad.
3	4	F	18	Good	Good	Excellent	Spastic Hemi.
4	10	M	6	Good	Good	Good	Spastic Quad.
5	6	F	7	Good	Good	Excellent	Spastic Hemi.
6	7	M	5	Fair	Good	Good	Spastic Quad.
7	3	F	3	Good	Good	No Problem	Mild Dipleg.
8	4	F	6	Good	Excellent	Fair	Spastic Para.
9	5	M	4	Good	Good	Fair	Spastic Para.
10	17	F	5	Good	Good	Good	Athetoid
11	5	M	5	Good	Good	Good	Athetoid
12	5	F	9	Fair	Good	Fair	Spastic Dipl.
13	3	M	12	Excellent	Excellent	Excellent	Spastic Quad.
14	7	F	10	Fair	Excellent	Good	Spastic Quad.
15	7	M	11	Good	Good	Excellent	Spastic Quad.
16	11	M	11	Good	Good	Good	Spastic Dipl.
17	4	M	10	Good	Good	Good	Spastic Dipl.
18	15	F	6	Poor	Fair	Fair	Spastic Dipl.
19	4	F	8	Excellent	Excellent	Excellent	Spastic Hemi.
20	7	M	8	Excellent	Excellent	Excellent	Spastic Hemi.
21	4.6 mo.	F	18	Excellent	Excellent	Good	Spastic Dipl.

Comments: Nos. 3, 13, 19, 20 and 21 no longer are required to wear the "skates" and are maintaining the correction they have achieved for periods of 6 to 18 months since removal.

Key to Improvement:
Poor—0 to 10 percent   Fair—10 to 30 percent   Good—30 to 60 percent   Excellent—60 to 90 percent

Patient number 21 was first seen two years previously when she was four and one-half years old. She was the oldest of two children, her sister being one year old at the time and normal in all respects. This patient was born blind and her problem was diagnosed as spastic quadriplegia. At the time we first examined her she could stand by herself for a very short period of time but could not walk without being held by the hand. She was very apprehensive and became alarmed at the slightest provocation. She held her feet in a very marked pigeon-toed position at all times and her limbs were always internally rotated. Upon examination we found that her limbs could be rotated externally about 40 degrees and internally 150 degrees.

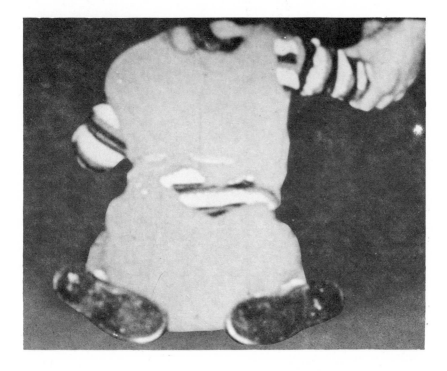

Fig. 118. Patient No. 21. Blind Quadriplegic Cerebral Palsy with Severe Scissors Gait and Spasticity. Note Feet in Crawling Position.

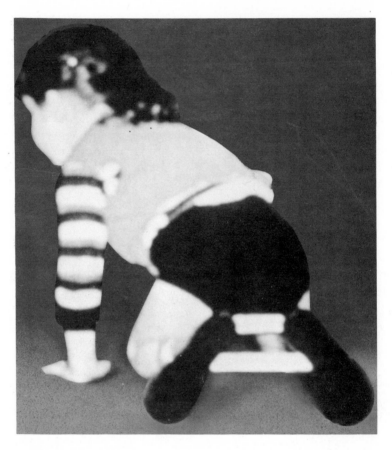

Fig. 119. Patient No. 21 with Skates Attached to Keep Feet in Outward Rotation.

The skates were constructed to maintain an external rotation of both feet and limbs at 30 degrees with a maximum external rotation of 90 degrees. The mother was instructed to keep the appliances on the child day and night and to remove them only when the child was bathed or dressed. After wearing the skates for eight months the child was allowed to go without them all day long but she wore them as a night splint.

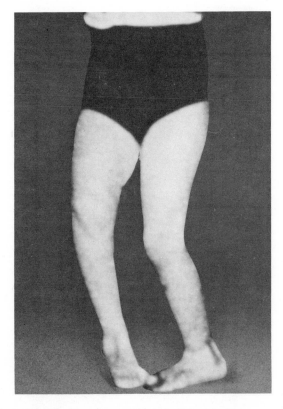

Fig. 120. Patient No. 21—Standing with Aid—Scissor's Gait.

In this patient as well as some others listed in the chart, we found that when the limbs were derotated and the feet were brought back into normal contact with the walking surface, a weakness in the longitudinal arch structures became evident. In each such instance we used supportive measures for the feet after the initial therapy had been completed. Our experience proved that balance therapy with the use of balance inlays provided adequate support. Two months ago this patient accompanied her mother on a shopping trip and visited our office the same day. Not only was her physical condition greatly improved, but her apprehensiveness and her entire outlook have benefited to a marked degree.

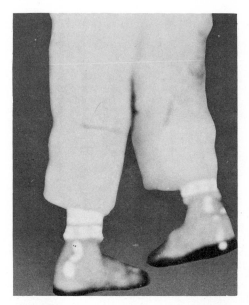

Fig. 121.   Patient No. 21—Standing Prior
to Treatment with "Skates."

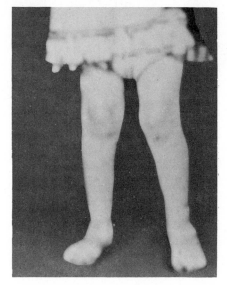

Fig. 122.   Patient No. 21—One year
after Treatment with "Skates."

Patient number 2 was three years and three months old when she was first examined. She was also diagnosed as a spastic quadriplegic and walked on her toes bilaterally with an inverted, or pigeon-toed gait. The left foot showed all signs of developing talipes equinovarus tendencies. This child, as well as patient number 21, had received exercises to stretch the posterior group of leg muscles for some time without positive results.

She wore the skates twenty-four hours a day and at the end of a two-month period her total gait was almost normal. At this stage the mother removed the skates during the period of warm weather and when the child was seen three months later some of the original symptoms had returned. The mother was instructed to keep them on full time for an additional three months before the child was allowed to remove the skates during the daytime. This follow-up program maintained full correction and the child did very well thereafter.

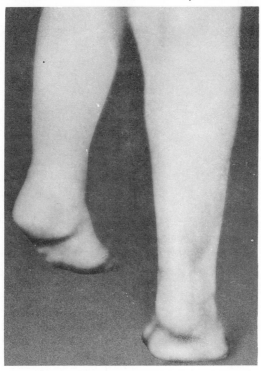

Fig. 123. Patient No. 2—Moderate Quadriplegic Cerebral Palsy. Note Equinus Gait before Treatment with "Skates."

Patient number 10 was a fully grown young adult, 17 years old, when she was first examined. She was attending high school for crippled children. A diagnosis of athetoid was made for this patient even though most of her actions were quite similar to those of a spastic quadriplegic. Her muscular structures were all tight and she exhibited a considerable amount of inco-ordinate motions. Her feet and legs rotated inward and she had developed a decided cross-legged or scissored gait. Both of her heels were elevated from the floor as she walked on her toes most of the time. Her standing balance was also awkward and unsteady.

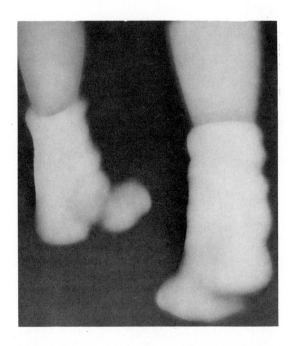

Fig. 124. Patient No. 10—Moderate Quadriplegic Cerebral Palsy—Female, Age Seventeen—Equinus Scissor's Gait—before Treatment with "Skates."

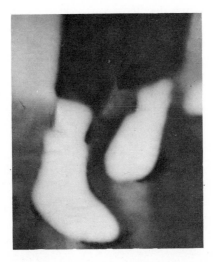

Fig. 125. Patient No. 10—Second View—before Correction.

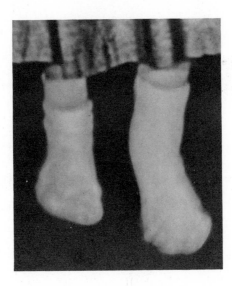

Fig. 126. Patient No. 10—Correction Achieved after Ten Weeks of Treatment with Skates.

In October 1955 we decided to use skate therapy on her because nothing further could be done for her condition. She was asked to wear them as much as possible and she cooperated very well. At school she removed them only when she had to leave the class to go home. On weekends she wore them full time. Good results were achieved with skate therapy in this young adult after ten weeks and maintained for a follow up period of two years.

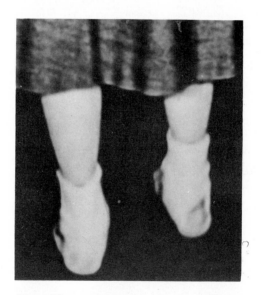

Fig. 127.   Patient No. 10—Second View
After Correction.

21. FOOT-RELATED DEFORMITIES OF THE HIP

CONGENITAL HIP DEFORMITY
Definition

There are many deformities affecting the lower extremities of children that must be thoroughly understood by the podiatrist even though it is not within his province to treat these deformities, and they may only come to his attention later in life when they create distinct foot problems. One of these deformities which may become very disabling in later life if it is not treated properly in its earliest stages is the congenital dislocation of the hip. The term dysplasia or hip dysplasia is sometimes used synonymously with the congenital dislocation terminology.

History

Dysplasia by itself means abnormal growth. Since a congenitally dislocated hip is abnormal in its growth, the terminology is quite proper. This condition was first described by Dupuytren in 1826. It was considered incurable until the year 1888 when Paci suggested the reduction of the dislocation. This reduction was popularized in 1895 by Lorenz. The incidence of this deformity is of considerable interest.

Prevalence

Congenital dislocation of the hip is five times as prevalent in girls as it is in boys. It appears twice as often in the left hip as in the right hip.

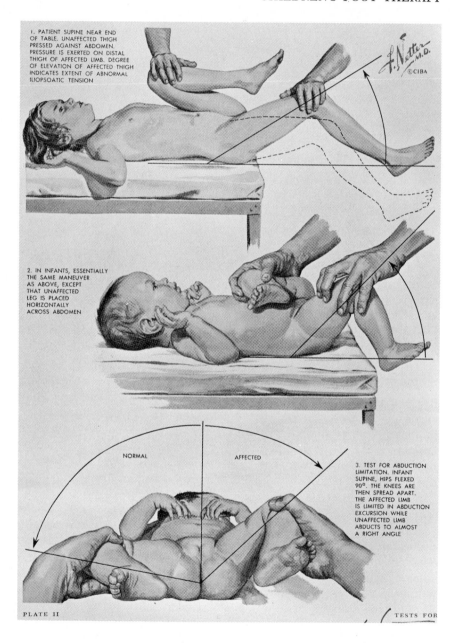

1. PATIENT SUPINE NEAR END OF TABLE. UNAFFECTED THIGH PRESSED AGAINST ABDOMEN. PRESSURE IS EXERTED ON DISTAL THIGH OF AFFECTED LIMB. DEGREE OF ELEVATION OF AFFECTED THIGH INDICATES EXTENT OF ABNORMAL ILIOPSOATIC TENSION

2. IN INFANTS, ESSENTIALLY THE SAME MANEUVER AS ABOVE, EXCEPT THAT UNAFFECTED LEG IS PLACED HORIZONTALLY ACROSS ABDOMEN

NORMAL   AFFECTED

3. TEST FOR ABDUCTION LIMITATION. INFANT SUPINE, HIPS FLEXED 90°. THE KNEES ARE THEN SPREAD APART. THE AFFECTED LIMB IS LIMITED IN ABDUCTION EXCURSION WHILE UNAFFECTED LIMB ABDUCTS TO ALMOST A RIGHT ANGLE

PLATE II   TESTS FOR

Fig. 128. By Permission of Ciba Pharmaceutical Co., F. Netter, M.D., from Clinical Symposia.

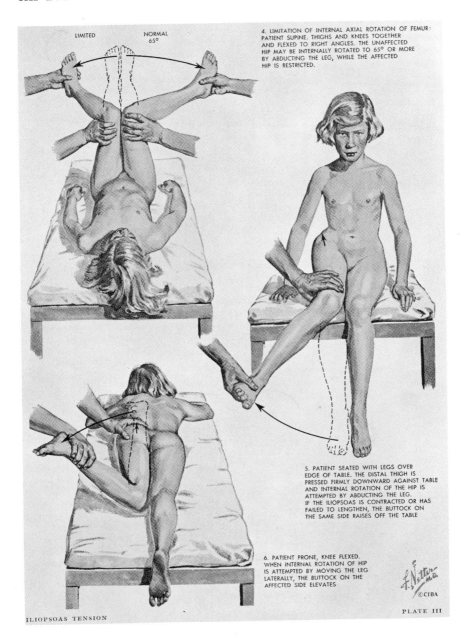

LIMITED

NORMAL 65°

4. LIMITATION OF INTERNAL AXIAL ROTATION OF FEMUR: PATIENT SUPINE. THIGHS AND KNEES TOGETHER AND FLEXED TO RIGHT ANGLES. THE UNAFFECTED HIP MAY BE INTERNALLY ROTATED TO 65° OR MORE BY ABDUCTING THE LEG, WHILE THE AFFECTED HIP IS RESTRICTED.

5. PATIENT SEATED WITH LEGS OVER EDGE OF TABLE. THE DISTAL THIGH IS PRESSED FIRMLY DOWNWARD AGAINST TABLE AND INTERNAL ROTATION OF THE HIP IS ATTEMPTED BY ABDUCTING THE LEG. IF THE ILIOPSOAS IS CONTRACTED OR HAS FAILED TO LENGTHEN, THE BUTTOCK ON THE SAME SIDE RAISES OFF THE TABLE

6. PATIENT PRONE, KNEE FLEXED. WHEN INTERNAL ROTATION OF HIP IS ATTEMPTED BY MOVING THE LEG LATERALLY, THE BUTTOCK ON THE AFFECTED SIDE ELEVATES

© CIBA

ILIOPSOAS TENSION

PLATE III

Fig. 129. By Permission of Ciba Pharmaceutical Co., F. Netter, M.D., from Clinical Symposia.

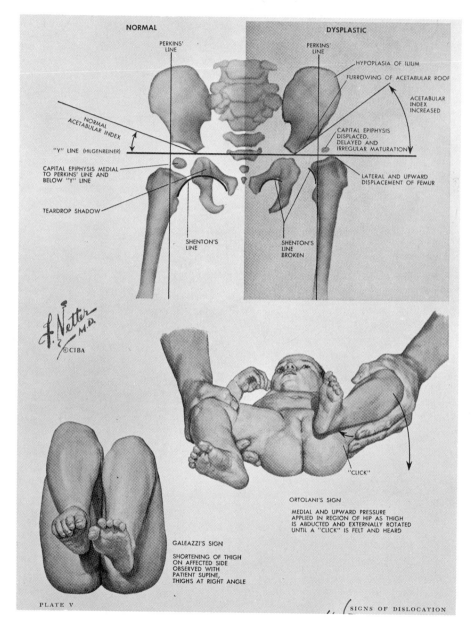

Fig. 130. By Permission of Ciba Pharmaceutical Co., F. Netter, M.D., from Clinical Symposia.

The deformity is present in much greater number with children in the northern states of the United States, and is quite common in the Latin races, especially in France and Italy. It is found infrequently in the Negro race. The etiology of congenital dislocation has not been generally established, but there are some factors that have been accepted.

Etiology

It is thought the primary developmental defect is associated with imperfect formation of the posterior-superior margin of the acetabulum in utero. There is excessive flexion and adduction of the hip in an abnormal uterus, causing stretching and lengthening of the hip joint ligaments. Some writers have attributed the deformity to an injury in utero. The heredity factor has also been given some significance because in one study of 1,900 cases thirteen per cent were found to be hereditary.

Pathology

Pathologically, congenital dislocation of the hip presents a number of changes that are easily recognizable. Early changes are minimal, but they increase with the duration of the dislocation. The deformity is usually divided into three segments. The first is known as pre-subluxation. At this stage, which is usually a very early stage, there is no displacement of the femoral head from the acetabulum. The second stage, known as subluxation, has a partial displacement of the head from the acetabulum, and the third stage, known as luxation, has a complete displacement of the head from the acetabulum.

Symptomatology

In the second and third stage particularly, the side of the ilium and the acetabulum becomes a straight line, and the cartilagenous rim of the acetabulum does not form. As the deformity progresses, the floor of the acetabulum fills up with fibrous tissue and is covered by the posterior and anterior surface of the capsule itself. Along with this, the acetabulum becomes very shallow. The normal hemispherical shape of the head of the femur becomes flattened and hammerhead-like, or conical, with a worn-away appearance. The neck of the femur is in the position of coxa vara, and is shorter than normal.

As time progresses and the condition is not treated properly, the capsule becomes the supporting structure of the joint, elongated and hour glass in shape. In time the muscles from the pelvis to the knee are shortened. This is particularly true of the gracilis, the head of

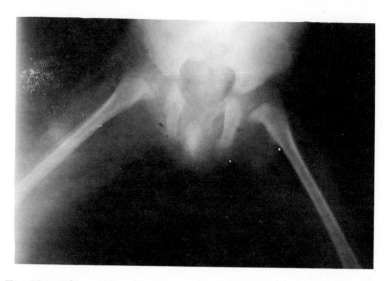

Fig. 131. Bilateral Congenital Dislocation—Three Month Old Female.

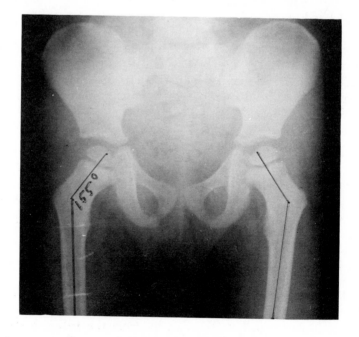

Fig. 132. Normal Hip—Three Year Old Female.

rectus femorus, and the sartorius. The muscles from the pelvis to the trochanter, however, are lengthened, and those primarily affected are the glutei, the soleus, and the quadratus femoris. A false acetabulum may develop as a furrow on the ileum; the pelvic tilt is normally sixty degrees with the horizontal, but in congenital dislocation it can become vertical and the entire side is tipped forward, causing marked lordosis and scoliosis toward the affected side in unilateral cases. No scoliosis is present in the bilateral problems.

Clinical Signs

The clinical symptoms associated with congenital dislocation of the hip are also quite evident upon examination, but they vary with each patient according to the degree of deformity. There is a click or snap of the hip on motion in the very young, and the jerk of entry and the jerk of exit. Both of these are known as Ortolani's signs. This jerk of entry and jerk of exit can be elicited upon manipulation of the hip itself, as the head of the femur enters and exits from the area of the acetabulum. There may also be a telescoping of the head of the femur if it fails to make contact with the nonexisting acetabulum and moves up and down along the side of the ilium.

When a luxation is present, it presents a very prominent femoral head which can be palpated. This is not common in the very young. Postural leg shortening is usually present and contraction of the adductor muscles, tendons, and ligaments represent a number of clinical signs. Among these are adduction and slight flexion attitude of the limbs, a rotational attitude of the limbs, asymmetry of the labial fold, the inguinal fold, and also the gluteal folds.

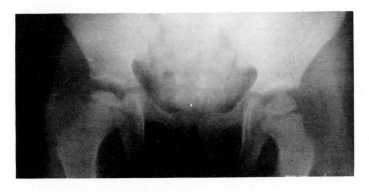

Fig. 133. Coxa Plana of Right Femoral Head—Three Year Old Female.

Diagnosis

There are extra and deeper adducter skin folds and creases and additional knee, popliteal and ankle creases. There is a definite obliquity to the pelvis and prominence of the lateral aspect of the hip. There is an absence of pain, inflammation, and muscle spasm. Since pain, inflammation, and muscle spasm are often found in other conditions associated with pathology of the hip, this makes a prominent point of differential diagnosis.

Roentgenologically there is an inhibited, delayed, and altered endochondral ossification of the innominate bone and femur with or without displacement of the femoral head from the acetabulum. Also, delayed ossification of the cartilagenous roof of the acetabulum which appears flat and inadequate. An altered and inhibited osteogenesis of the femoral head is present. Acetabular dysplasia may persist while femoral head dysplasia improves, or vice versa, but pelvic obliquity and adduction of the extremities are constant observations.

Treatment

Two types of treatment are used for the correction of congenital dislocation of the hip. These are generally classified under the terms "closed reduction" and "open reduction." Although there is no unanimity of opinion as to the greatest value of each of these methods, it is generally conceded that closed reduction should be tried first and at the earliest age possible. Most authorities believe that if closed reduction is attempted in the very early stages, that is, within the first few days or the first few weeks of life, most congenital dislocations can be corrected before the child is three months old.

The treatment of choice seems to be the use of Ortolani's maneuver to bring the head of the femur back into the acetabulum or the acetabular position and to follow this with the use of a Frejka pillow properly applied and retained for a period of weeks or until the condition is symptomatically corrected. If the condition is treated properly, the hips and the limbs are held in an abducted and flexed position with the feet adducted.

If the child is three months or older before treatment is begun most of the problems are treated by casting the legs and hips in the frog-leg position, with the hips and legs abducted and flexed but with the feet somewhat internally rotated and inverted. The cast is reapplied every two to six weeks, depending upon the problem and treatment is continued for a period of two to six months after the cast is removed. The limbs are usually held in an abducted position with the feet internally rotated. This is accomplished by the use of a bar attached to the soles of the shoes. The best type of spreader action is obtained if the bar is from eighteen to twenty-four inches long and fixed in the shape of a bow.

Children who have not had the benefit of early treatment and where the deformity has reached the stage of luxation, usually receive very little benefit from the closed reduction treatment. In these children the open reduction appears to have the best chances of bringing about the proper corrections.

In many instances, as a child grows older and considerable correction has been achieved, a residual foot problem remains. This may take a number of forms. There may be a structural shortage causing a limp, there may be a smaller foot size as a result of atrophy of the entire extremity, or there may be an associated weakness in all of the muscular structures of the limb and foot. As a result, there may also be bony changes and changes in the digits resulting in digital deformities. Many of these patients seek attention and must remain under the constant supervision of a podiatrist for the remainder of their lives.

Wilk reports on an extensive study of 186 children with 204 diseased hips which were diagnosed as juvenile osteochondrosis of the hip. His etiological findings do not differ much from those of other observers except for the fact that he found spina bifida occulta was present in most cases. Of this finding, Wilk writes: "An interesting finding that did evolve from this study was the incidence of spina bifida occulta, especially of the first sacral segment. This abnormality may or may not indicate an underlying neurological problem. In most patients spina bifida occulta was diagnosed as an incidental finding. The exact incidence of spina bifida occulta is not known, but it is thought to be about twenty per cent in asymptomatic patients. Nevertheless, the occurrence in the present study is fairly high and probably significant." Further study of this relationship is required. Wilk's investigation has included only non-operative treatments. Wilk believes that complete bed rest is an excellent form of therapy and agrees with the view of many other observers in this regard, however, he states that it is an almost impossible task for the parents to keep these youngsters in bed from one to three years or more. He prescribes such treatment only for the most cooperative parents and patients. For most of his patients he uses a type of ischial weight bearing calipers which enables the child to go to school and to carry on in a fairly normal capacity. It must be pointed out, however, that many authorities disagree with Wilk's opinion that this is the best form of treatment.

LEGG-PERTHES

Definition

Another hip deformity which may come to the attention of the podiatrist who treats a number of children in his practice is Legg-Perthes' disease. Other synonyms used for Legg-Perthes' disease in the literature are coxa plana and osteochondritis deformans coxa juvenilus. A simple definition would be a disease of the hip characterized by a slight limp and little or no pain and limited by age and sex, with resulting changes in the femoral head.

Etiology

The problem is usually found in children from three to ten years of age, and in the incidence we find that of those affected, eighty percent are males. It is also noted that ninety per cent of those affected have unilateral problems. Legg-Perthes' disease is responsible for ten to fifteen percent of all hip cases seen in children. Although there is no unanimous opinion of the etiology of the Legg-Perthes' problem, most authorities believe that an untreated synovitis of the hip due originally to respiratory illness, trauma, or allergic manifestations is a primary causative factor. This brings about an inflammation at the hip joint with a low-grade infection. It is also believed that the etiology may be due to a thyroid deficiency or to vascular interference in the head and neck of the femur.

Pathology

The course of Legg-Perthes' disease has been clearly established and is well understood. There are three stages to the disease. The first is the incipient stage which lasts from two to four weeks. In this stage roentgenologically there may appear a swelling of the capsular shadows and a widening of the joint space with osteoporosis of the femoral metaphysis in the neck adjacent to the epiphyseal line. In the second stage there is an aseptic necrosis, and this stage may last from one to two years. This includes all of the changes of the first stage, together with an increase in the density of the areas of the femoral head and irregularity in the epiphyseal line. The third stage is the regenerative stage, which may take from three to four years. Here radiopaque areas begin to appear and since considerable mechanical malformation may have taken place, there are abnormal anatomic outlines. In this last stage, regeneration of the head is complete but the end result may be that of a coxa magna or sometimes a coxa plana.

Some general statements relating to the pathology can be made with reference to these three stages. At the beginning there is a thickening of the capsule and synovium, with an increased thickness of cartilage of the femoral neck and head. The synovium becomes edematous and hyperemic, and the metaphyseal area may be softened by increased vascularity. The femoral head undergoes necrosis and then fibrous tissue replacement. In the healing process, bone again replaces the fibrous tissue areas.

Clinical Signs

The clinical picture also is of considerable significance. There is generally a history of limping, and some pain in the knee of three weeks' to two months' duration. Hip flexion on the affected side and contracture is elicited. There is a limitation of internal rotation and abduction with the knee and hip flexed. There usually is some tenderness on palpation, anterior and posterior to the hip joint. Associated with this, there may be an atrophy of one-half to one inch at the mid thigh, and only occasionally will there be some acute distress. In most instances, pain is not one of the primary factors associated with the clinical picture in this disease.

Differential Diagnosis

In considering differential diagnosis we must think of tuberculosis of the hip, rheumatic fever, and rheumatoid arthritis. A fourth consideration must be slipped femoral epiphysis. However, in each of the conditions listed, there is usually an association of severe pain, a generalized or marked rise in body temperature, a limitation of motion associated with an inability to bear weight, and all of these generally add up to a child who is not active in any sense of the word.

Treatment

Certain pertinent factors must be considered in treatment of Legg-Perthes' disease. The head of the femur must be protected from mechanical forces that will flatten and widen it. Full joint motion must be maintained to the greatest degree possible. A strict program of non-weight bearing must be maintained for a period of time, usually fixed at a minimum of one year and followed by a nonweight-bearing splint until full recovery has been achieved. A return to weight bearing is justified when there has been no new dense area formed in the femoral head for at least two months after the roentgenograms have shown normal bone formation in the head of the femur, and the patient must also have full motion at the hip joint.

There are two primary reasons why the podiatrist should take a very active interest in Legg-Perthes' disease in children. (1) the first symptoms develop with an early limp and a limited amount of pain, which many parents associate with foot problems and the child will be brought into the office of the podiatrist for examination. One of the simple functional tests that is always used in our office is to have the child hop on one leg. It is readily understandable that if there is a joint problem present in the ankle, knee, or the hip, the child will not be able to hop effectively on the involved side, and further examination will therefore be conducted to determine where the pathology exists. When Legg-Perthes' disease is suspected, the child should be sent to a medical orthopedist who is trained to handle these problems adequately.

Children who are cared for properly usually have no further complications after the hip has healed, but there are many instances where the joint does not heal adequately and there is a limitation of range of motion at the hip which may be associated with a generalized limb shortage, limb weakness, and an inadequate position of the foot and leg in general for proper weight bearing. This brings about a variety of foot problems that come to the attention of the podiatrist, and, again, may require the services of the podiatrist for many years. In our office we have found that in congenital hip conditions and in Legg-Perthes' disease mechanical therapy affords the greatest amount of relief for these patients who are left with some residual problems.

Erlacher, states that the best results are expected when treatment is begun within the first six months of life. The discussion centers on the use of the harness designed by A. Pavlik, an orthopedic surgeon from Czechoslovakia, which permits children with dysplasia of the hip to achieve self reduction through their natural movements. This apparatus consists of straps that reach down to the heels and embrace them stirrup-like. The straps are suspended on a harness in such a manner that the knee and hip joints are held in ninety degrees of flexion. Of 300 out-patients, some treated by the author, ninety-eight per cent achieved self reduction. After a few years of observation ninety-four per cent appeared clinically and roentgenographically normal.

22. SYSTEMICALLY - RELATED FOOT PROBLEMS

Most parents bring their children to the podiatrist with the complaint that the posture or gait is faulty. The child does not usually complain of pain in the feet except where there is a skin tumor present such as a verruca or where injury has taken place. Whenever a child complains of pain for any other reason, we must conduct a very thorough emamination to rule out all systemic problems that may be the basis for the pain. Etiologically, pain may be the result of an infective problem, a glandular condition, or neurological; it may have some vascular implications or associated with one of the muscular deficiencies which are prevalent but not thoroughly understood. There may be times when foot and leg pains are associated with metabolic disturbances because many children react quickly to food and liquid intake which can be disturbing to the digestive system of the body.

The following case history will demonstrate quite clearly how recurring pains in the feet can be overlooked by both the physician and the podiatrist: On the twenty-second of July, 1963, a six-year-old, white male was brought to the Foot Clinics of Chicago by his mother with complaints of pain in both feet. Several weeks previous to this visit the patient suffered a sudden pain in the left foot which was so severe that the child could not walk and was put in bed. The family physician was notified and the child was promptly hospitalized. A series of blood tests and X-rays were taken and rheumatic fever and rheumatoid arthritis were ruled out. The physician arrived at a diagnosis of inflammation of the deep veins and the child was dismissed from the hospital under the care of the physician.

The following day the right foot became very painful and this episode of pain lasted for three days. On July seventeenth the left foot was similarly affected with the pain subsiding after two days. On July twentieth the right foot again became very painful. The patient was brought to the Foot Clinics on July twenty-second.

The history elicited from the mother indicated that the child had had measles and a twenty-four hour virus infection. A physical examination did not suggest any condition of a systemic nature. Since this child walked with an intoeing gait and the radiographs revealed a moderate pes adductus, the diagnosis was one of compensatory forefoot adduction associated with rear foot weakness. All neurological signs appeared to be normal. Mayo pads were placed in the shoes and the patient was asked to return after one week. On July twenty-ninth, four days following the first visit, the patient was brought back to the clinics complaining of an attack of pain in the left foot. Examination revealed arthralgia of the ankle joint, talonavicular joint and erythema, elevated temperature, edema and excessive perspiration associated with the entire left foot. Oral temperature was 101.8. Anorexia and extreme fatigue of the patient was observed.

The patient was referred immediately to a pediatrician for further consultation. After some exhaustive tests the pediatrician made a diagnosis of endocarditis and rheumatic fever. In reviewing this case it was observed that the primary findings were recurrent pains in both the left and right foot. Again we must stress that recurring pains in both feet and legs must be given the most careful consideration and in all such instances systemic conditions must be considered. When pains of this nature occur proper consultation is mandatory.

MICRODACTYLIA

Under the subject of systemic conditions manifesting themselves in the feet, we must consider microdactylia of the great toes. In most instances where microdactylia of the great toe is present, it is a positive sign of progressive myositis ossificans which is a disorder of the mesodermal tissues in which scattered inflammatory foci first appear and proliferate in fibrous tissue such as the intramuscular fascias and the tendons and ligaments. In the early months after birth and the early years, the lesions are largely confined to the neck and trunk and the extremities are relatively or absolutely free. While this hypoplasia of the phalanges of the great toes is present, the metatarsals are entirely normal in size and appearance.

VON RECKLINGHAUSEN'S DISEASE

Among the less common problems affecting infants and children is Von Recklinghausen's disease. This disease is generally known as one of the degenerative diseases called osteitis fibrosis cystica. It is a localized fibrocystic disease of the bone wherein there is a fibrous transformation of bone marrow by an unknown agent. It is sometimes known as fibrous dysplasia.

Pathology

The lesion is usually multiple with fusion symmetrical enlargement of the bone and thinning of the cortex. The cancellous bone is replaced by firm yellowish white tissue which contains small cysts filled with fluid, and the principal component of the lesion is connective tissue arranged in bundles within which are found trabeculae of newly formed bone.

Radiographic Findings

The first changes found in X-rays is in the metaphysis of the long bones. The areas of translucency become confluent and the process extends to the diaphysis, then to the entire bone.

Clinical Signs

The initial sign is local swelling and tenderness. Very often the shaft of the tibia alone is involved with the upper end of the tibia showing the bone cystic formations. Pathologic fractures are common in this condition and they heal on immobilization.

Treatment

The treatment depends on the site of the lesion and prognosis is often good where thorough curettage can be done bone destruction is not excessive when the disease is discovered. Recurrence may be encountered. In most instances the greatest protection is obtained with braces used for prolonged periods of time. Foot care is important at all stages of this disease because of the strain imposed on the feet as a result of the problem in the lower extremities.

OSTEOMYELITIS

Prior to the discovery of antibiotics one of the most serious bone problems affecting children was acute osteomyelitis. This problem is not so prevalent at the present time but it does occur with sufficient frequency to require a considerable understanding of its implications.

Predisposing Causes

The disease is found primarily in infancy and childhood and is prevalent in males over females at the ratio of four to one. The primary etiology is thought to be trauma because usually there is a history of direct blow to the part. The location of the injury is usually at the metaphysis of the long bone and in many instances the upper end of the tibia and the lower end of the femur are affected. Poor nutrition and poor hygiene are also thought to be attending factors and sometimes there is an antecedent focus of infection either in the tonsils or from boils.

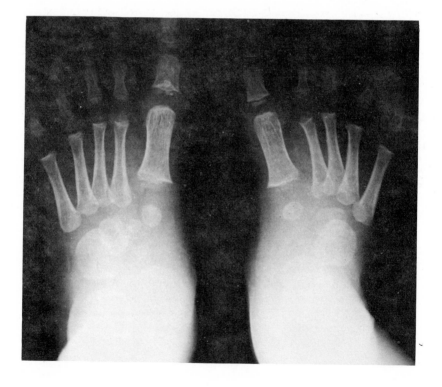

Fig. 134. Talipes of Right Foot with Splay Foot Resulting from Osteomyelitis of Femur.

Exciting Causes

The most common organism found in osteomyelitis is hemolytic staphylococcus aureus. Streptococcus is found less commonly and other organisms are rare.

Pathogenesis

Septicemia or bacteremia is usually present and an infective embolus enters the nutrient artery and is trapped in a vessel of small caliber. It is known that the longer and larger bones are more susceptible to acute osteomyelitis than the small bones and because there are fewer phagocytes in the metaphysis the area offers excellent culture media. The involved organisms block the small vessels and a small area of the bone becomes necrotic. As a result of this hyperemia demobilization, pain develops and the surrounding bone becomes decalcified. The resulting compression destroys other tissues in the area and the exudate follows along the subperiosteal spaces with the infection spreading along fascial planes. The osteomyelitis becomes chronic when the walled off areas of the infection become symptomatic at any time in later years.

Clinical Signs

At the onset all symptoms of severe acute illness appear. The child is restless, complaining of headaches; there is vomiting, chills, and convulsions may take place. There is also a high fever with a rapid pulse rate and a 30,000 white count. The extremity is usually held in semiflexion and the surrounding muscles are in spasm with passive motion resistant because of pain. At first there is no swelling, but in a few days the affected site becomes red and edematous. If the infection and septicemia continue unabated, this problem can be fatal.

Laboratory Findings

The X-rays may be negative for the first ten days but later show wide zones of decalcification of bone at the metaphysis. After a few weeks periosteal shadows become elevated and later a moth-eaten appearance includes the medulla. Aspiration in this area will supply a subperiosteal pus which reveals infecting organisms and blood culture demonstrates bacteremia. The blood count will include polymorphoneuclear leukocytosis.

Complications

If the infection spreads into the soft tissues it may cause suppurative tenosynovitis, suppurative arthritis, and thrombophlebitis.

Differential Diagnosis

The condition may simulate rheumatic fever except for the fact that in rheumatic fever the onset is more gradual and constitutional symptoms are less acute. Pain and tenderness in rheumatic fever are also less acute and the involvement is usually polyarticular and migratory, not limited to one small area. In rheumatic fever the response to salicylates is dramatic while antibiotics have no effect.

Ewing's tumor may also be considered in differential diagnosis. In this tumor, however, the destruction is usually confined to the diaphysis and not the metaphysis. Ewing's tumor involves a more diffuse area of infection and it responds rapidly to X-ray radiation. The constitutional symptoms are less acute and a biopsy shows typical tumor cells.

Another differential diagnosis may be acute suppurative arthritis. However, in this condition the fluid accumulation in the joint occurs early and pain and tenderness are limited to the joint itself. Joint movement is greatly restricted. Muscle spasm is intense and aspiration reveals purulent synovial fluid.

Prognosis

Antibiotics have reduced the mortality rate from twenty per cent to near zero. The infection can be cured rapidly by antibiotics in the early stages and the small areas of necrotic tissue and bone may be reabsorbed and normal bone architecture restored.

Treatment

Antibiotics given immediately in large doses and continued indefinitely bring best results. Drainage is important very early and all supportive treatment is essential. Where treatment is inadequate or not begun early enough the results often cause a considerable amount of disability in the lower extremities associated with structural shortages. In the past we have seen many sequelae of acute osteomyelitis and occasionally we still are called on to take care of the foot problems resulting from this disease. In general, most of these problems relate to shortages and limitations of motion in the ankle or foot joints. Oftentimes this precipitates a talipes equinovarus with a marked rigidity at the ankle joint and the foot in plantar flexion. The construction of the proper mechanical devices to establish more normal weight bearing is the treatment of choice.

23. METABOLIC HYPOTHYROIDISM

One of the most interesting foot findings related to metabolic factors in children is hypothyroidism which affects the feet of children more frequently than suspected. This is especially true with children whose X-rays reveal a delayed appearance of the tarsal and other bones. It is known that there is a correlation of thyroid function with delayed osseous development of all bones, including the midtarsal bones, and particularly the navicular and cuneiforms. When laboratory tests are taken and blood cholesterol elevation is associated with this delayed osseous development, we must think of hypothyroidism. The feet of these children are usually quite flat in appearance, with fatty pads on the dorsum and short toes. There will be a positive Helbing's sign and most of the symptoms of so-called "weak foot." The general posture of the child is poor, with a protruding stomach, weak musculature, easily broken nails, crowded and decaying teeth, and a slow pulse.

When the mother is questioned relative to the child's activity, she will usually offer the information that the child is irritable, unable to play actively for any length of time because of the short attention span, poor concentration, restlessness during the night, and there may be an associated enuresis. These children are usually hard to get up in the morning and groggy. During the day they tire readily, and, if they can be made to rest for a time, they appear refreshed after the rest. It has been thought that the hypothyroid child is always obese, but this is not true because there have been many cases where these children are actually underweight. Children with these symptoms require thyroid therapy and in association with this they should also be given calcium, preferably in the form of calcium lactate, which is the most soluble form of calcium for maximum absorption. Calcium lactate can be given in citrus juice thirty minutes before breakfast very effectively in doses of one to two teaspoons. Calcium lactate wafers are also available.

The use of mechanical therapy alone is not effective when treating these children. It is entirely possible that many children who have not responded to the use of metal therapy fall into this classification.

HYPERADRENIA

Another condition similar to this is hyperadrenia which may sometimes be confused with that found in the hypothyroid individual because some of the symptoms are similar. The clinical signs associated with the syndrome of chronic mild adrenal cortical hormone insufficiency must be recognized. These are primarily characterized by pronated ankles, slumped posture, easily broken nails, and increasing perspiration of the palms and the soles.

It is said that these patients perspire so freely when under nervous tension that during examination they may leave small puddles of perspiration on the table beside them. Stiffness and tightness in the neck and back ligaments are often associated with this problem, and these patients also tire very easily. This is especially true of children because they become emotionally unstable when fatigued and develop temper tantrums during this time. Corrective exercises alone to support the pronated ankles in these children are not effective because the muscles are just too tired to do the work effectively for any length of time. Therapy includes adrenal cortical extracts in addition to corrective exercises.

OBESITY

Another metabolic factor associated with foot pain and hormonal disturbances is obesity. It is well known that obesity can cause a good deal of foot distress by the wear and tear that is produced on the foot and its surrounding structures as a result of the excess weight that is constantly thrust upon these structures. The very best treatment for obesity, no matter what the cause, is a high-protein, low-carbohydrate diet. It is said that patients who follow this dietary program gradually lose weight and their appetite for carbohydrates as well.

RICKETS

While rickets is considered to be a rare disease at the present time, facts disprove this contention. It is true that we do not see many children

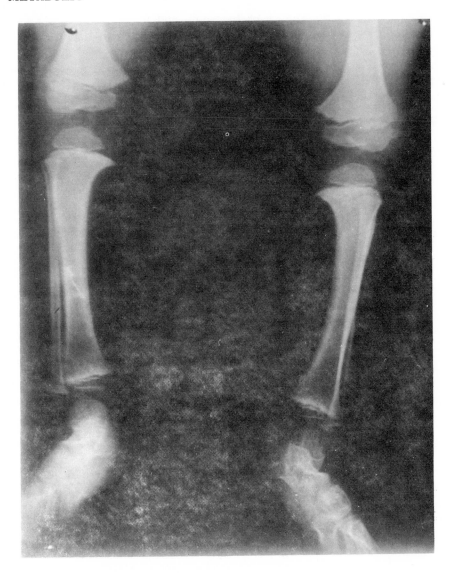

Fig. 135. Rickets—Eight Year Old Male. Note Flare of Long Bones.

with the marked deformities of the spine and lower extremities that have been caused by rickets in the past, but there are a considerable number of children who have rachitic tendencies and some problems in the spine and lower extremities that can be traced to this disease of infancy. For this reason we should consider rickets as one of the childhood diseases that must be understood and dealt with.

Definition

By definition, rickets is a disease of infancy and childhood due to deficiency of vitamin D and characterized clinically by softened and deformed bones.

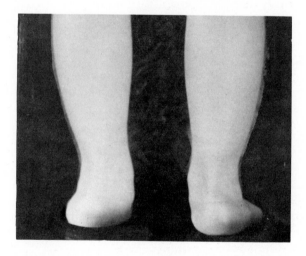

Fig. 136. Pes Planovalgus—Rachitic Patient in Fig. 136.

Etiology

The abnormal ossification is due to a vitamin D deficiency associated with intestinal diseases and a dietary lack of calcium and phosphorus. Some information concerning vitamin D is important to understand. Vitamin D promotes absorption of the minerals from the intestines. It is fat-soluble and is usually associated in foods with vitamin A. Vitamin D is found in its strongest concentration in fish liver oils and is present in lesser quantities in milk, cream, butter, egg yolk and animal fats. It may also be prepared commercially by irradiation of ergosterol, a yeast lipoid. Untraviolet rays of the sun or mercury quartz lamp converts steroids in the skin to vitamin D while dust, window glass and skin pigmentations would impede the penetration of the ultraviolet rays.

Intestinal diseases may be involved. The celiac disease, sprue, and common diarrhea cause their effect in one of three ways: Fat is inadequately digested and combines with calcium and phosphorus to form soaps which are eliminated. Vitamin D, being fat soluble, is also elminated and intestinal irritation reduces absorptive powers.

Insufficient calcium and phosphorus implies a diet consisting of foods with minimal amounts of these minerals. Milk, cheese, nuts and cabbage contain an abundance of calcium phosphate and should be used. Rickets is rare during the first six months of life because of the ample nutrition of the child when in utero. However, prenatal calcium and vitamin deficiency in the mother is a main cause of the form of rickets known as fetal rickets or osteomalacia. Infantile rickets, is most common between six months and three years of age. There is a separation of the epiphyses, especially of the upper femur. The disease occurs mainly in the winter months when there is less sunlight, especially in nontropical regions. Negro and Italian races show a marked predisposition to rickets.

Pathology

The histological feature of rickets and osteomalacia is osteoid tissue in which calcium and phosphorus salt has failed to deposit. This process is divided into two stages: In the active stage the orderly progression of enchondral ossification is interrupted at the epiphyseal plate. The formation of the matrix is normal but calcification of the matrix is deficient. An enormous accumulation of proliferated cartilage and osteoid tissue results in a widened, irregular epiphyseal line which is radiolucent and the rachitic rosary at the costochondral junction of the ribs is seen in children and infants.

The second stage is the healing stage. Calcium salts are deposited in the ones of preparatory calcification. The capillaries penetrate the area of proliferated chondrocytes and deposit bone tissue about the calcified cartilage. The thickened epiphyseal plate is reduced to normal size and normal bone architecture appears. The bone extremities often become corrected spontaneously.

Symptoms

First, there is a history of dietary deficiency, with increased rest-lessness at night and profuse diaphoresis. There is a skin pallor and a disinclination to play normally. The child has generalized catarrh of the mucous membranes with frequent diarrhea and respiratory infection. There is an irritability of the central nervous system known as hypocalce-mia producing spasms and often convulsions.

Clinical Findings

The head is enlarged and square in appearance and the fontanels are late in closing. The bones are thin and crackling. The chest shows beading enlargements at the costochondral junctions and with hori-zontal depressions a few inches above the lower costal margin. The breast is known as pigeon-breast. The abdomen is prominent and the pelvis inlet is narrowed. There is an enlarged epiphysis at the knees and the wrist bones and dentition is delayed. There is skin pallor which is second-ary to anemia. Poor muscle tone is very prominent and there are de-formities such as knock-knees, bowlegs, coxa vara and lax ligaments. Incomplete fractures are frequent. Growth is restricted in general.

Roentgenographic Findings

The ossification center in the epiphysis is poorly defined and smaller

than normal, and the epiphyseal border of the metaphysis is cup-shaped, ill-defined and frayed. This is particularly true at the lower end of the femur and the upper end of the tibia. The metaphyseal cortexes flare outward.

Treatment

Vitamin D and exposure to sunlight are the primary treatments. Calcium preparations are also used and active treatment will reverse the disease beginning with the second week in which treatment is initi-ated.

CONGENITAL ABSENCE OF FIBULA

Congenital absence of the fibula is a rare condition which has been described by a small number of orthopedic men during the past twenty years. In all, approximately 100 patients have been listed with this condition. Most authors consider the etiology of the condition is ob-scure, although there is some thought that the defect is an acquired anomaly resulting from an accidental injury to the embryo at about the sixth or seventh week. One of the authors, Ingalls, believes that anoxia within the embryo may be a primary factor. The term used to describe the condition is "congenital absence of the fibula," but there are other problems associated with this deformity. Not only is the fibula absent, but there is usually some tibial bowing, associated with a growth deficiency in the extremity, and foot deformities. In one of our patients, a three-year-old boy, there was an absence of the fibula in the left leg, together with a bent tibia, a fusion and malformation of the talus and calcaneus, and three metatarsal shafts with three digits on each foot. The left foot was held in a talipes equinovalgus position, and the right foot in a talipes equinovarus position, as can be observed from the X-ray illustrated above. The boy in this illustration has been walking for the past year and one-half. The gait was very awkward, but he was able to balance himself, though he took frequent falls. After some attempt at correction of the valgus and varus deformities, the child was referred to the orthopedic section at Mayo Clinic for surgical correction.

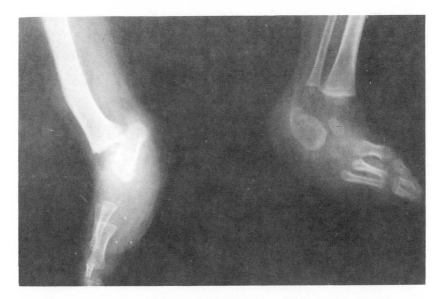

Fig. 137. X-rays of a Three Year Old Male with Absence of Fibula and Bent Tibia Right Foot. Talipes Equinovalgus, Right—Talipes Equinovarus, Left—Three Metatarsals and Toes Each Foot.

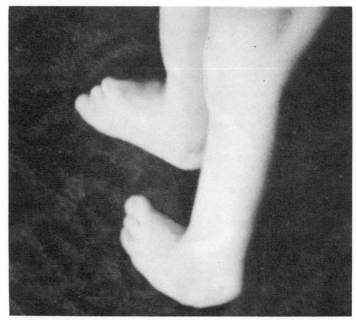

Fig. 138. Side View of Feet—Patient Fig. 138.

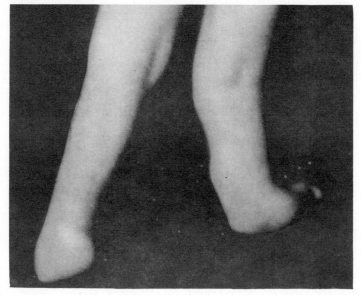

Fig. 139. Rear View.

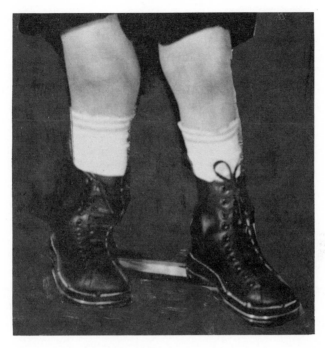

Fig. 140. Patient Above Wearing Skates in Attempt to Effect Some Correction.

24. FOOT RELATED DISEASES OF SPINAL ORIGIN

PERONEAL MUSCULAR ATROPHY

Peroneal neuropathic musclar-trophy, also known as hereditary muscular atrophy, and Charcot-Marie-Tooth disease is occasionally seen in younger children.

Etiology

While the cause is unknown, the disease is known to be transmitted as a dominant recessive of sex linked characteristic and it is predominantly found in males appearing between five and ten years of age.

Pathology

The degenerative process takes place without inflammation. Primary locations are at the anterior horn cells, the posterior columns and peripheral nerves. The pathology is limited to the somatic muscles with atrophy of some muscle fibers and swelling of others and increase in connective tissue symptoms. There is also a deposition of fat between the hypertrophied membranes of the muscles.

Clinical Picture

These children develop clumsy gaits with ankle inversion strains which are thought to be due to the peroneal weakness. The legs develop some pain and paresthesia with a gradual atrophy of the leg muscles and intrinsic foot muscles. There is an equinovarus deformity and a clawing of the toes. A steppage gait results and becomes progressively worse in some instances. The greatest weakness is reflected in the peroneal and the tibial muscles. Associated with this is a loss of deep reflexes and a loss of tactile, temperature, and proprioceptive senses, primarily in the lower extremities. The face, trunk, pelvic and shoulder girdle are not affected. Considering all of the problems, drop foot may be the most incapacitating in time. There is also an impairment of the vibratory sense.

Prognosis

The course is slowly progressive but may become arrested at any time and the disease has no effect on the life span of the patient.

Treatment

Prostigmine bromide given in dosages of 15 mg. t.i.d. may lessen the weakness and the ataxia. In the early stages spring drop-foot braces are sometimes used and in some instances surgery has been advocated and used, with varying degrees of success. We have found that all of these patients require the use of balance therapy with the addition of shoe therapy whenever necessary.

FRIEDREICH'S ATAXIA

A synonym is hereditary spinal ataxia. This is an hereditary disease characterized by progressive degeneration of corticospinal, spinal, cerebellar and posterior columns of the spinal cord.

Etiology

Although the etiology is unknown, the onset usually begins at ten years of age and may be transmitted through affected and unaffected parents.

Pathology

Demyelinization occurs in pyramidal tracts, spinal, cerebral tracts and posterior columns. The disease may affect the anterior horn cells.

Clinical Picture

There is an awkward gait at onset. Stumbling, frequent falls and frequent turnings of the ankles may be present. Foot pains and fatigue are generally present and shoes become very uncomfortable. Bilateral clawfoot with marked elevation of the longitudinal arches and prominence of the metatarsal heads appear. There is a widening of the forefoot with muscular weakness in the peroneals and anterior tibial muscles.

Prognosis

This is a slowly progressive disease over many years and the gait becomes ataxic. Rhomberg sign becomes positive and a dyskinesia develops. The deep tendon reflexes are lost early. Deep pain, position, and vibratory senses are impaired attesting to a posterior column lesion. Later pyramidal tracts become involved and reflexes become hyperactive and an extreme equinovarus deformity may develop and may become very disabling. The patient may become bedridden at thirty with a kyphoscoliosis as an additional deformity.

Treatment

After full bone growth has taken place surgical intervention may be of some help and brace therapy is often used with some success.

SYRINGOMYELIA

This is a slowly progressive disease of the spinal cord and medulla oblongata caused by cavitation and gliosis and characterized clinically by memory loss and muscular atrophy.

Etiology

The cause is unknown. It may be a developmental anomaly or it may be secondary to vascular lesions, lues, tumors of the spine and trauma to the cord. It is more common in males and develops from ten to thirty years of age.

Pathology

The primary involvement is to the gray matter at the center of the cord in cervical and lumbar areas, and it spreads upward to the medulla and down to the thoracic area as fluid finds paths of least resistance. When the fluid invades the anterior horn cells, the pyramidal tract of posterior columns it produces atrophies, spasticity and ataxia.

Prognosis

The disease is slowly progressive and may become stationary at any time.

Treatment

The primary treatment is drainage of the cavity. When this is successful the condition is usually arrested.

PROGRESSIVE SPINAL MUSCULAR ATROPHY

This disease is characterized by progressive weakness and atrophy of the muscles of the hands and arms first, then the lower extremity.

The etiology is unknown.

Pathology

The cervical spinal cord is involved and the entire cord becomes affected. The anterior horn cells degenerate, disappear and are replaced by glio tissue.

Clinical Findings

The symptoms appear insidiously at middle age and are most often found in males. At first there is weakness in the use of the hands, with very little or no pain. There are no deep reflexes involved and the sensations remain intact.

Prognosis

The development of this disease is slow and protracted, sometimes taking 25 years before it is complete; it is not fatal.

FAMILIAL PROGRESSIVE SPINAL MUSCULAR ATROPHY

A synonym is Werdnig-Hoffmann disease. This is a rare form of progressive degeneration of the anterior horn cells. It is familial and the onset of flaccid paralysis occurs at early infancy. The disease generally terminates in death at five years of age.

AMYOTONIA CONGENITA

The synonym for this disease is Oppenheim's disease. This disease is due to a failure of the anterior horn cells in the lower half of the spinal cord to develop. There is a flaccid paralysis with absence of deep reflexes. The disease may improve with the passage of time. We have had several infants and young children referred to us with this disease for foot care. In every instance, the application of balance inlays or metal braces has been helpful in getting these children to walk with a fair degree of normalcy. In one instance of a three-year-old child the application of Roberts plates enabled the child to walk for the first time after the plates were applied. She was not able to initiate weight bearing prior to that time because of the marked collapse at the ankles.

AMYOTROPHIC LATERAL SCLEROSIS

In this disease there is a rapid progression of degeneration of the anterior horn cells in pyramidal tracts, involving both spinal cord and brain stem. It occurs in middle-aged males who develop a weakness, atrophy and flaccid paralysis in the upper extremities and spastic paralysis in the lower extremities. The atrophy involves all muscles. The disease is rapidly progressive and death occurs in two to five years.

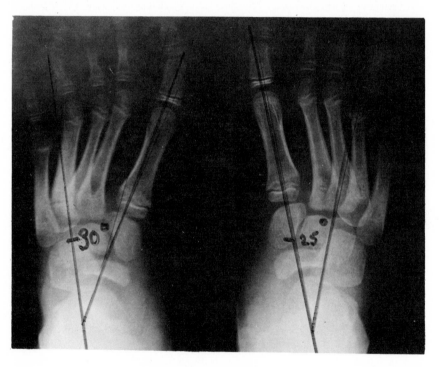

Fig. 141. X-ray of Seven Year Old Male with Spina Bifida Oeculta and Associated Talipes Equinovarus.

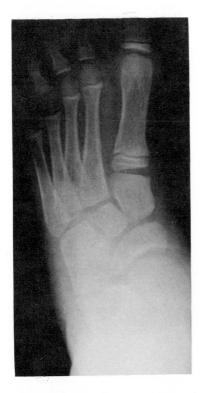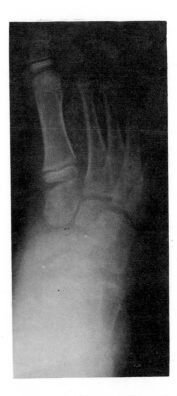

Fig. 142. X-ray of Patient in 142 at Age Twelve—After Use of "Skates" for Two Years.

POLIOMYELITIS

Poliomyelitis, or infantile paralysis, has plagued the children and young adults of the world, but with the advent of the Salk vaccine we now see very few victims of poliomyelitis. The etiology is now known to be a filterable virus, but the portal of entry is still unknown. The disease was primarily prevalent during the warm months and all races and classes were affected. Pathologically, there is a cellular infiltration and congestion of the posterior ganglia, and the posterior nerve roots may be responsible for the severe peripheral neuritis accompanying this disease. Efferent nerve fibers from the destroyed neurons degenerate and the muscles which they formerly enervated atrophy and become fibrotic. The lower extremities were particularly susceptible to this disease, and quite often one single muscle such as the anterior tibial became completely paralyzed without any apparent changes in other muscles entering the foot. In many other instances all of the muscles of the lower extremity became paralyzed; in other words, there was no specific pattern to the paralysis of the muscles of the lower extremity. In many instances the end result of the paralysis was a flail foot, with no stability whatever at the ankle. In order to be able to walk, these patients required positive mechanical therapy such as foot and leg braces and in some instances only foot plates which would immobilize the relationship between the foot and the ankle.

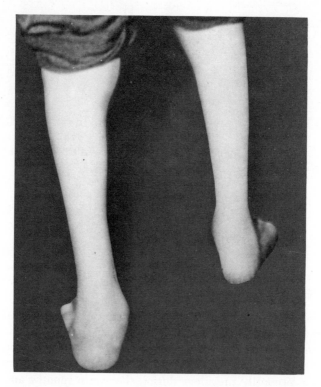

Fig. 143. Marked Muscular Atrophy of Posterior Muscle Group in Lower Limbs of Thirteen Year Old Male with Pes Valgus.

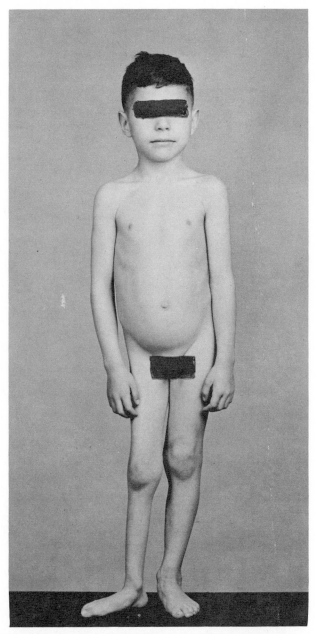

Fig. 144. Post Polio in Eight Year Old Male—Left Limb Involvement. Note
    Severe Postural Changes.

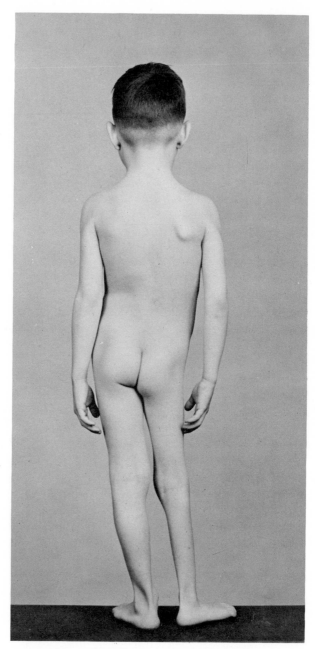

Fig. 145. Same Patient as 145—Rear View.

Low Voltage Currents

There are times in the application of low voltage currents to patients' extremities will bring about a single specific movement no matter where the electrodes are attached. This is possibly related to the dominance of the reflexes mentioned. It has been stated that whenever we find such dominance present, we should use every means possible to overcome that dominance and thereby avoid the difficulties that may ensue at some later date.

There are some neurological problems which may require an electromyographic examination and a measurement of nerve conduction velocity. Such an examination should be conducted by those who are expert in carrying out the examination and in recording the findings. Physiatrists have done a considerable amount of work in the last number of years in the development of this type of testing.

Congenital Absence of Coccyx—A Case Report

John N. was eighteen months old when he was brought to our office. His birth history was insignificant, but his mother observed the lack of normal motion of the lower extremities from the time he was one month old. At three months of age a diagnosis of hip dysplasia was made and from that time until John was fourteen months old he wore a Frejka splint. John could never crawl nor was he able to pull himself up to his feet in the crib.

It was observed that his toilet habits were very irregular and there was some question as to whether he was incontinent.

At fourteen months, the mother became concerned about his progress because of his inability to walk and also because of some deformities that were apparent in his feet.

With a full realization that John had a congenital hip problem, we took X-rays of the hips. These X-rays revealed that John was born without a coccyx. At this stage we called in an orthopedic surgeon and John was taken to a hospital for further observation and study. The study revealed that John had a severe spinal cord problem. He was not receiving the innervation required to his sphincters and the entire sciatic nerve was involved in the activation of his lower extremities. The muscles in John's thighs were fairly normal, whereas all of the muscles below the knee and entering the foot were almost rudimentary and had little power or function. As a consequence, his range of motion was also abnormal. He had a limited amount of dorsiflexion and plantar flexion, but could not initiate abduction or adduction. John's reflexes were almost totally absent in his lower extremities. The boy was placed in a spica cast from his feet to his waist and his legs were held in a frog-leg position.

His feet were inverted and gave the appearance of a talipes equinovarus. We constructed a bar which was attached to the cast to hold his feet in an everted and abducted attitude. When the casts were removed after three months, there appeared to be a fairly consistent development in the region of the acetabulum and the feet were held in a good position for the beginning of weight bearing and walking. At this stage John was fitted with some Roberts plates of stainless steel inserted into shoes which held his feet and ankles in the normal attitude. Thereafter, John was encouraged to stand as much as possible and within several months he began to take a few steps.

By the time John was two years of age he was able to walk with a wide spread stance in a somewhat hesitant attitude. The following year the boy improved his walking to some degree. He was considerably undersized for his age and he remained undersized for years.

The next five years the child was seen every three months. When he was six or seven years old, we discarded the Roberts plates and constructed balance inlays for his feet. At this stage the inlays were worn in high Keds and John appeared to function fairly well in consideration of his basic problem. The boy remained incontinent and since he could never be toilet-trained, it was difficult for him to adjust himself to going to school, but he finally made the adjustment and he got along quite well because he was not handicapped mentally. When John was nine years of age a urologist attempted to repair the sphincter control for his bladder and rectum. This surgery was almost fatal for John, but he did recover after a period of about six months and the results of the surgery were only fair.

At the present time John is twelve years of age and still under our care for his foot and leg problems. His feet are somewhat reminiscent of those of a child with a severe pes plano valgus problem, but he has very little or no movement in his toes and still no ability to abduct or adduct at the ankle. There is a limited amount of dorsiflexion and plantar flexion, just as there was when John was a year and a half old. Muscular development below the knees is very inadequate, but there is sufficient power for the boy to get about at school and play without any assistance.

During all of these years John has had the closest attention to his footgear and his appliances. We believe that it is this supervision that has enabled him to remain on his feet. We also believe that John will be compelled to have foot care for the remainder of his life.

CASE REPORT—CHARCOT-MARIE-TOOTH DISEASE

About 15 years ago two brothers, Phillip and Robert M., were brought to our office for evaluation of their foot problems. At this time Robert was fourteen years old and Phillip was ten. The family had a long history of Marie Strumpell's disease and both boys had been affected at birth. When Robert was eight years old he had a triple arthrodesis performed on both feet. Phillip, whose foot problems were equally severe, did not have surgery. Phillip's feet have the typical high arches that are generally found with the condition. All of the digits were contracted and the tendons on the dorsum of the foot were very prominent. There was a marked limitation of dorsiflexion bilaterally with some limitation of plantar flexion. Both the peroneal muscles and tibal muscles were also quite weak.

On weight bearing it was quite noticeable that most of the weight was borne on the calcaneus and the ball of the foot only. The findings of the left foot were primarily those of pes cavus; the right foot could be described as that of a talipes equinovarus because there was a considerable prominence at the base of the fifth metatarsal and the forefoot was inverted to a marked degree. Phillip walked with somewhat of a steppage gait and as may well be understood, the right foot was held in somewhat of a varus attitude with most of the weight bearing being initiated on the lateral margin.

Because of the triple arthrodesis that had been performed several years earlier, Robert walked with a stilted gait because he could initiate no motion in any of the joints below the ankle except for slight motion at the metatarsal-phalangeal articulations.

There was a considerable difference in the leg structure of Robert and Phillip. Robert showed marked atrophy in the area of the calf, while Phillip showed good development of his muscular structures in this region. In spite of the fact that Robert had had a triple arthrodesis on both feet, both boys complained of early fatigue and foot pains and aches, especially when they were required to remain on their feet for any considerable length of time an examination of Robert's feet revealed excresences under the first, third and fifth metatarsal heads and on both the fifth toes, which were painful. Phillip had no excresences.

Because both brothers exhibited a distinct lack of normal weight-bearing area on both feet, we decided to make balance inlays for both so that we might increase the weight-bearing surface and at the same time redistribute some of the excessive weight on the heels and balls of both feet. The appliances achieved this primary objective and as

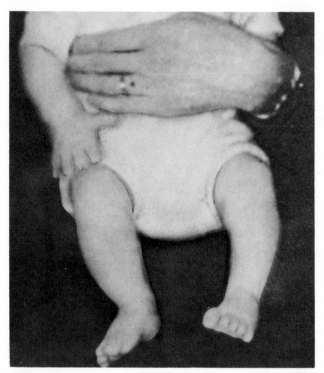

Fig. 146. Patient Robert M. Holding Son Age Three Months—Talipes Equinovarus is Apparent.

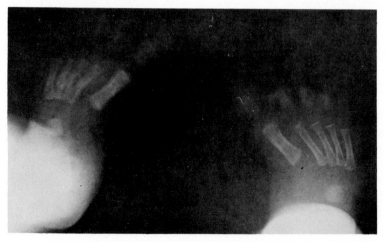

Fig. 147. X-rays of Patient Above. Note Varus Forefeet.

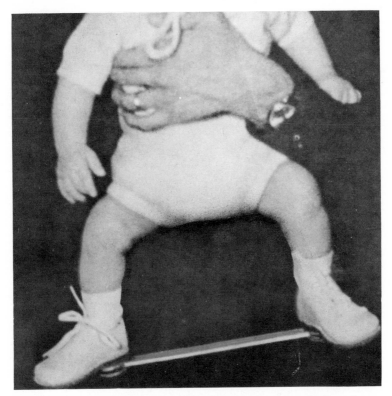

Fig. 148. Patient in Fig. 157 with Shoes and "Skates" Attached in Corrected Position.

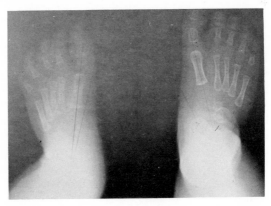

Fig. 149. Patient Above Showing X-rays after Four Months of Treatment with "Skates.

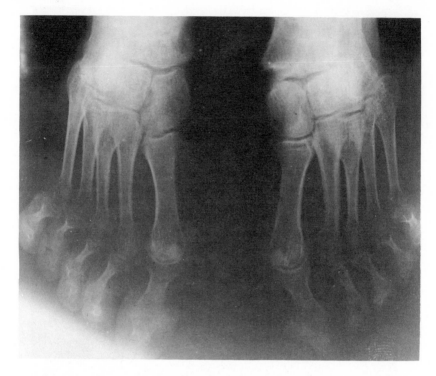

Fig. 150. Dorso-Plantar X-rays of Robert M.

they wore out or changed with growth of the feet, we replaced them with new appliances over the fifteen-year period since we first observed these two boys.

About three years ago Phillip married and a son was born one year later. When the infant was three months old the pediatrician observed that both feet were assuming the talipes equinovarus position and instructed the parents to have something done about this problem immediately because he was aware of the condition of the father and other members of the family. The infant was brought in for my observation and we detected all of the cardinal signs that are associated with a talipes equinovarus problem, only the X-rays did not show the malforma-

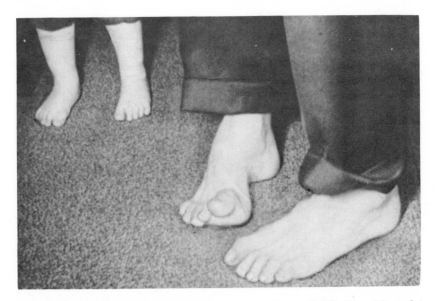

Fig. 151. Photos of Robert M. and Son at Age Two. Child's Feet Normal in
        Appearance and Function.

tions of the talus and calcaneus that usually accompany a talipes
equinovarus. It was decided to place the child in skates, which we fixed
in the abducted position, for a period of twenty-four hours a day. The
infant wore these devices day and night for sixty days. After this time,
the wearing period was reduced two hours a day for the next three
months. At eight months of age the devices were removed for daytime
wear entirely and the child wore them only at night.

He began to stand and walk at twelve months and at fourteen
months the skates were eliminated entirely. This child is now three
years old and all further examinations have demonstrated a complete
correction of the talipes equinus position.

In comparing the feet of Phillip and Robert at this writing fifteen
years after we began our initial treatment with both boys, we must conclude that Phillip, who has had no surgery, functions better and has
less difficulty than his brother who had a triple arthrodesis.

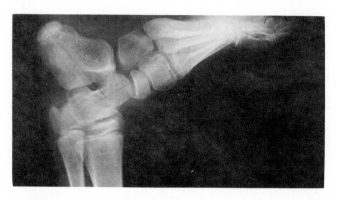

Fig. 152. Friedrich's Ataxia—Medial Lateral X-ray—Young Adult.

CONGENITAL AMPUTATIONS

Congenital amputations are also known by the terms of anomalies, spontaneous intrauterine amputations, congenital constricting bands, spontaneous amputations, and congenital annular defects. While the etiology is unknown, some authors including Lewin suggest that it may be due to pressure on the fetus in utero, while Pillay and Hisketh contend that it may be hereditary occasionally. These investigators have also found that in thirty-seven and five tenths per cent of the congenital amputations they have seen, clubfoot was also present. The degree of severity of these congenital amputations may vary from mild to very severe.

There may be just superficial circumferential grooves in the skin, and there may also be an amputation of the entire limb or part of the limb,. In the lower extremity, most of these defects occur below the knee, usually in the toes and the foot itself. Cowan gives an excellent nomenclature and description of the conditions, and follows up with his terminology.

McKeever states that the relationship between short legs and static scoliosis and between pronation of the feet and lordosis is generally known. However, few medical men recognize visceroptosis, rounded dorsal kyphosis, and forward projection of the head as being caused by faulty weight bearing. He further states that the form and structure of the foot at birth are hereditary, and that spontaneous correction of pseudo deformities produced by position in utero does not occur. In other words, when these deformities do exist, they must be treated. According to McKeever, there are at least twenty-seven accessory bones in the foot, and only one, the accessory scaphoid or the supernumerary navicular, is associated with weak foot and marked pronation. It is his contention that this supernumerary bone does not cause the pronation, but defective ligamentous architecture and a mechanical disadvantage which accompany it and its supporting tendons usually result in marked pronation.

25. SYSTEMIC RELATED
PROBLEMS OF GROWTH

ACHONDROPLASIA

A synonym of achondroplasia is chondrodystrophy foetalis. This condition is considered to be hereditary and is characterized by a normal size trunk but with short upper and lower extremities. Because the primary cartilage of the limbs and the epiphyseal cartilage fails to proliferate normally, its effect is a diminished growth in length of the upper and lower extremities. Individuals with this problem are recognized as achondroplastic dwarfs. Their hands very seldom reach their hips when hanging down at the sides. Lordosis of the back and a prominent forehead are usually in evidence, and the fingers are short and stumpy. The mental development does not necessarily have to be impaired. In most instances achondroplastic dwarfs walk with a marked outward rotation and a severely pronated foot results. Because of their poor posture and under-developed lower extremities, there is a certain amount of postural instability. As children they require a considerable amount of attention in order to prevent further foot problems resulting from the pronounced out-toeing. These patients do well with periodic foot care for the remainder of their lives. Most of the foot care is prophylactic in nature.

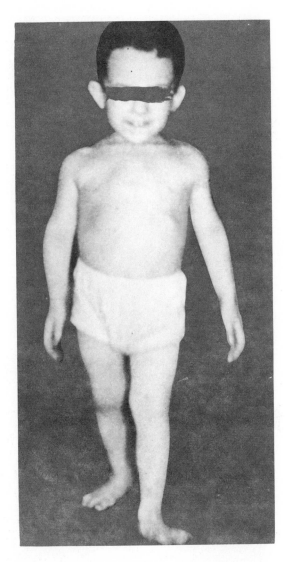

Fig. 153. Achondroplastic Dwarf—Age 9. Note Marked Foot Abduction and Pes Planovalgus.

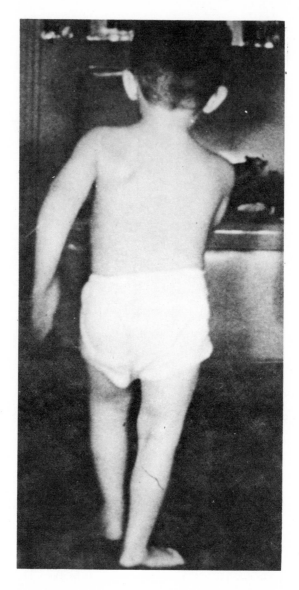

Fig. 154. Rear View of Patient Fig. 153. Arms Swing Widely for Maintenance of Balance.

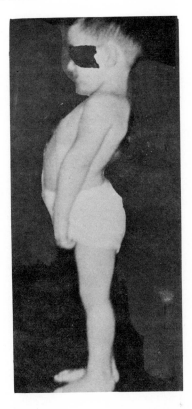

Fig. 155. Side View of Patient Fig. 153. Note Severe Kyphosis of Sacro-Lumbar Area of Spine.

ARACHNODACTYLY

Arachnodactyly patients are recognized primarily by a marked elongation of the long bones of the hands and feet. A synonym for this condition is spider digits. Marfan's syndrome is also thought to be related to this condition. These patients have very little subcutaneous fat, and their muscles are hypoplastic and hypotonic in nature. Because of the great elongation of the long bones in the feet and the loss of subcutaneous fat in associated tissue, these patients present feet that are pes planovalgus in appearance and less than adequate in muscular

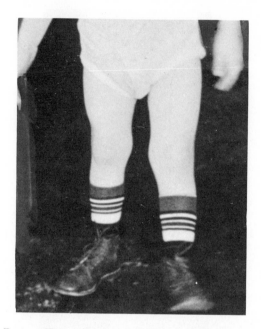

Fig. 156. Same Patient Fig. 153 after One Year of Treatment with "Skates." Marked Correction of Abduction.

quality. There is also a considerable amount of ligamentous weakness through the mid-tarsal area of the feet. When this condition is diagnosed in early childhood, it is best to use supportive measures such as appliance therapy to maintain the foot in the proper position and relationship to the ankle and the superstructure. Wherever this condition is associated with systemic diseases such as congenital heart disease, it is important to stress systemic care by the family doctor.

ARTHROGRYPOSIS—Two Case Reports

During the past twenty years, five of these children have been referred to our office for foot care and gait training. All of these children had a pronounced talipes equinovarus condition. In every instance the knee joints and ankle joints were enlarged and the muscles were small, hypotonic and weak. Tendon reflexes were all absent. There was a limited degree of active and passive motion, but always sufficient motion to induce some weight bearing and walking.

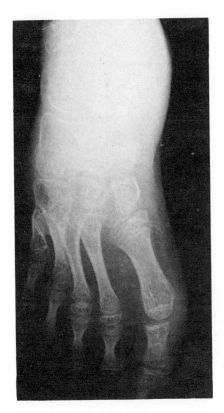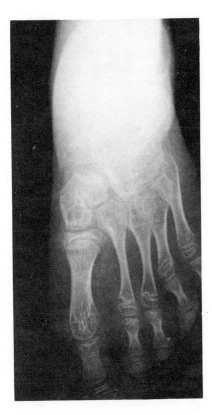

Fig. 157. Tommy L.—Dorso-Plantar View. Note Pathology Present in Metatarsal and Mid-tarsal Bones. Demineralization is Prevalent in All
Long Bones. Right Leg Is Three Inches Short.

Tommy L. was eleven years old when first referred to our office. At
a very early stage, Tommy had more than twenty surgical procedures
performed on his joints in the upper and lower extremities. These sur-
geries were necessary to prevent distortion and deformity.

An examination revealed that Tommy walked with a marked pigeon
toed gait. He had an approximately four inch shortage on the left side
and although he walked with a considerable limp, he got along fairly
well considering the amount of deformity present.

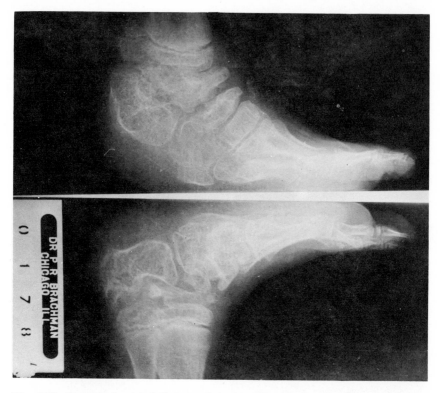

Fig. 158. Tommy L.—Medial Lateral View—All Tarsal and Mid-tarsal Bones
    Are Mal-formed.

Examination of his feet revealed a severe talipes equinus deformity
bilaterally. His ankles were enlarged and his knee joints were also
quite large despite the fact that he had had extensive surgery. There
were a number of scars from the surgery, including those of a triple
arthrodesis performed on both feet. He had had rotation osteotomies on
both legs through the tibias and fibulas, yet Tommy still walked with
a marked inverted gait. The surgeon who referred him to our office
was in hopes that we could eliminate this attitude in weight bearing.
With this inversion, Tommy walked on the outer margins of his feet
and if this were continued for a long period of time, it would have
made the triple arthrodesis practically useless. We decided to apply
skate therapy, and by the derotation of his limbs at the hip joints, we
hoped that it would be possible to overcome the attitude of internal
rotation.

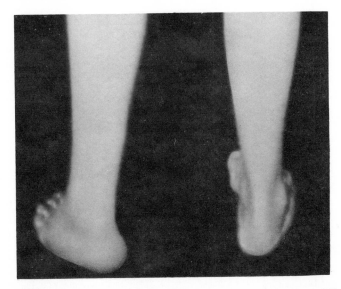

Fig. 159. Tommy L.—Posterior View before Use of "Skates" to Effect Derotation.

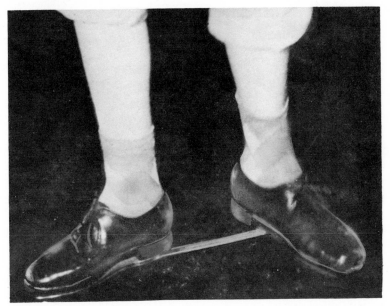

Fig. 160. Tommy L.—Wearing Shoes with "Skates" Attached. Worn for One
Year, Eight Hours Every Day.

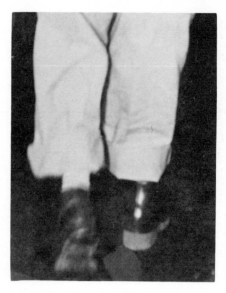

Fig. 161. Tommy L.—After Correction Wearing Shoes with Three Inch Elevation of Right Heel and Sole.

Tommy could not perform this outward range of motion himself because the muscles were not functioning in his lower extremities; only a change in the relationship at the hip joint where there was a possibility of stretching muscles, ligaments and the capsule might bring about the correction required.

The boy was fitted with the proper surgical shoes and the skates were attached. He and his family were instructed that he was to wear the skates constantly for twenty-four hours a day for the next three months. Though Tommy lived a considerable distance from our office, we did see him every two weeks during this period to make certain that there were no complications.

At the end of three months we were surprised to see the amount of improvement in the internal rotation problem. At this time Tommy walked with a slight amount of abduction and we had high hopes of correcting this condition within the following three months.

In order to make ambulation easier, a four inch elevation was placed on the shoe of the short limb. This elevation was built up with a synthetic rubber material so that the procedure was inexpensive and very functional.

During the second three months, Tommy wore the skates for only eight hours a day. We made some balanced inlays for his feet to be placed into another pair of shoes, and again the shoe for the short limb was built up four inches.

We saw Tommy every three months for the following two to three years, and during all this time the changes that had been produced by the use of the skates remained without any deviation.

About this same period, Mary K. was referred to our office with the diagnosis of arthrogryposis multiplex congenita. Mary was six and one-half years old. She also had a number of surgical procedures on her upper and lower extremities. Among the procedures were a bilateral triple arthrodesis, bilateral exterior tendon transplants and Achilles tendon lengthenings. Mary K., however, did not have any rotation osteotomies. Despite the triple arthrodesis, the talipes equinovarus tendency was still present and she walked with a severe amount of inversion. There was a marked limitation of motion in all planes of the foot and leg. The hip motion was fair and there was a poor muscular development in both legs. Mary walked on her toes with a waddling gait. We applied skate therapy and asked the parents to make certain that she would use these skates for twenty-four hours a day for the next three months.

Because Mary K. lived approximately 300 miles from our office, it was not possible for her parents to bring her in every two weeks. However, we did see her once a month for the first three months. It became quite apparent after the first visit that the parents were not insisting that Mary wear the skates the full twenty-four hours a day, because the results that we noted were not consistent with the type of results that should have been achieved had the instruction been carried out properly.

At the end of three months, it was still apparent that the instructions were not being carried out to our satisfaction. Mary still walked with an inverted gait of approximately twenty degrees but her toe walking was lessened and her waddling gait had been improved. The parents were then asked to carry out the same program for the next three months.

At the end of six months there was some additional improvement, but the results were not as satisfactory as those we had achieved on the boy just described. We continued to use the skates on Mary K's

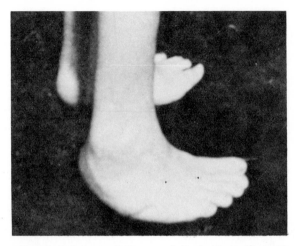

Fig. 162. Mary K.—Medial Lateral Views of Both Feet. Note Convexity of Lateral Margin.

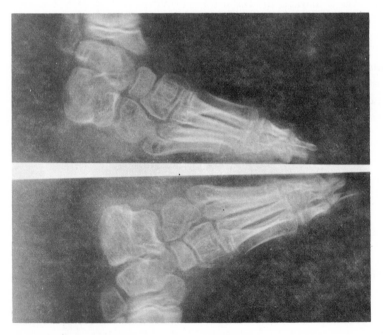

Fig. 163. Mary K.—Medial Lateral X-ray Views.

shoes for the next two years. It was necessary to allow the parents to use their own judgment when the skates were going to be used, because it was not possible to force the issue with them.

The last time we saw Mary was when she was approximately nine years old. At that time she walked with a slight adducted gait but her heels were down and the waddling was not too noticeable. Although we had not achieved the type of correction that we would have desired, the parents were well satisfied with the results.

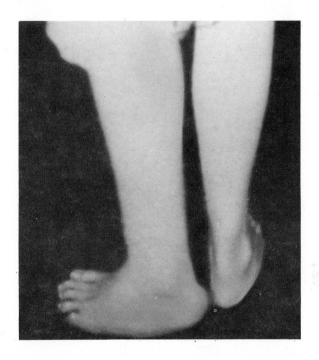

Fig. 164. Mary K.—Limbs Outward Rotated after Correction for One Year.

OSTEOGENESIS IMPERFECTA

Common synonyms for this problem is brittle bones, and fragilitas ossium. This is considered a hereditary condition characterized by the fragility of bones of the extremities, often of the bones of the trunk itself. Pathologically it appears that the formation of bone by the periosteum and the formation of osteoblasts are defective. Many fractures may appear in the bones at birth, and if these children survive, the tendency toward fracturing lessens and the possibility of survival is quite good. An adolescent type is sometimes present where the fractures result from minimal trauma but as the children grow older this tendency diminishes and may be outgrown with time. Supportive measures applied to the feet can do nothing but good; in fact, where the fractures occur in the feet along with other areas of the body, proper appliances and shoes may avoid some of the trauma which may occur if no attention is given this factor.

26. DISEASES OF MUSCLES

Diseases of the muscles may be divided into those that affect children, either in early or later childhood, and those that affect adults primarily.

MYOTONIA CONGENITA

Myotonia congenita, also known as congenital myotonia and Thomsen's disease, is considered to be hereditary but the first symptoms may not occur until the child is six to eight years of age. The primary symptom relates to a defect in the ability to relax the muscles promptly after an initial forceful contraction.

Pathologically there is no degeneration seen and the central nervous system is not involved. Biopsy will not reveal any exceptional lesions other than a hypertrophy of all muscle fibers. Males and females are affected equally. Myotonia and pronounced muscular hypertrophy are the cardinal symptoms manifested in this disease during childhood. Similar to children with cerebral palsy, the child with this disease may not be able to roll over or hold its head erect or walk until a date much later than the average child.

While the muscles of the lower extremity are primarily affected, the disease may affect all skeletal muscles of the body. The patient finds that it is difficult to initiate movement at the beginning but after repeated movements, a rapid relaxation will occur; then, upon rest again, movements become slow and they are accompanied by muscle spasm. A change in the type of activity, such as a change from walking to climbing stairs, will also produce difficulties. Certain movements

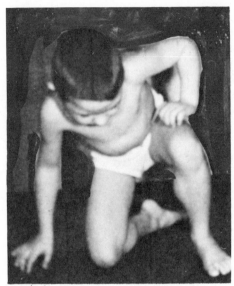

Fig. 165. Six Year Old Boy with Pseudo-hypertrophic Muscular Dystrophy.
Child Attempts to Arise from Sitting Position and Finds It Almost
Impossible To Do So. Patient Becomes Fatigued with Very Little
Effort.

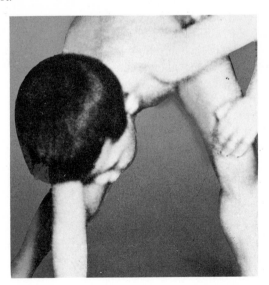

Fig. 166. Same Patient Attempting to Arise by Supporting Himself by Stabiliz-
ing Knee.

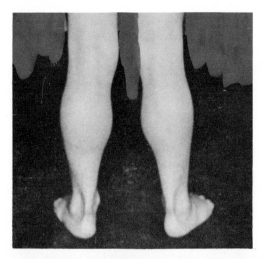

Fig. 167. Same Patient Exhibiting Marked Hypertrophy of Calf Muscles.

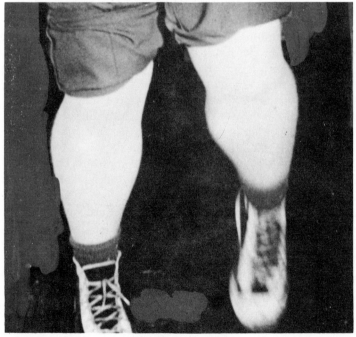

Fig. 168. Same Patient at Eleven Years of Age. Note Marked Additional Hypertrophy. Patient Now Spends Most of His Time in Wheel Chair. Progressive Deterioration.

may set up an involuntary spasm of the whole limb which might be more powerful than the original movement and incapable of modification by the patient.

The condition may become aggravated by exposure to low temperatures, emotional excitement, and prolonged rest. Quinine appears to have some beneficial action, as does calcium and Vitamin C. Because of the involved problem, specific foot care is not particularly indicated. Most of these patients require generalized prophylaxis for their feet.

DYSTONIA MUSCULORUM DEFORMANS

Dystonia musculorum deformans is described as a rare disease of the basal ganglia in which dystonia beginning in the neck, arm, or foot, may spread to the trunk and other limbs and bring about a considerable distortion of the whole body, especially the extremities. The pathology is neurologic, with the thalamus and parts of the cerebral cortex being primarily affected. The disease usually begins in childhood, between the ages of six and twelve, and may start with a spasmodic inversion of one foot or inclination of the head to one side. Rest may bring about some relaxation but the spasm may gradually become more continuous and involve additional muscles. The contraction of the opposing muscles to the spasm can result in great distortion of the ankles, spine, and hands. Tendon reflexes are present. In this disease the prognosis is bad, and there is no known satisfactory treatment.

Amyotonia congenita, also known as Oppenheim's disease, is characterized primarily by a weakness and flaccidity of the muscles of the body, and appears either at birth or during the first few months of life. Pathologically it is due to a degeneration of the anterior horn cells associated with the retardation of motor development. Because the muscles are flaccid, there is a marked hyperextensibility of the joints, but no paralysis is present even though the tendon reflexes are absent. The legs and the feet are affected in every case, the arms in ninety per cent of the cases, and the facial muscles in about thirty-three per cent. Infants may find it difficult to sit up and walk at the normal age but appear mentally unimpaired. These are instances where disease does not progress and many patients show improvement as time goes on. However, it is generally thought that the outcome is unsatisfactory and the prognosis is fatal, although there have been cases where patients have survived to adulthood. In these cases there is such a marked pronation and collapse of all of the ligamentous structures of the ankle that infants and young children find it difficult to bear weight. In treating several patients with this condition, we have found that the use of high shoes and balance inlays have the effect of giving them sufficient support so that they may begin walking before two years of age. Proper foot care is of considerable value in this condition.

Calmenson states that in a survey of medical literature a great deal has been written about rehabilitation of the handicapped child in recent years but there is a dearth of literature restricted to those who have only a foot handicap. According to a study reported by Calmenson, there are 3,168,000 persons with physical disability restricted to orthopedic impairments in the United States. Since there are no accurate statistics as to the distribution of these physical disabilities with relationship to the foot, we can only estimate that a good number of these listed are for foot defects. Handicapped children must endure many problems of adjustment during their lifetime. It is essential for the podiatrist to take his place with the other members of the health team to help the handicapped child in every area possible.

BIBLIOGRAPHY

Bennet, G. A., Wayne, E. and Bauer, W.: Changes in the Joint at Various Ages and Particular Reference to the Nature and Development of Degenerative Joint Diseases, New York, Commonwealth Fund Report, 1952.

Bersani, Frank A.: "Massive Familial Tarsal Synostosis," Journal of Bone and Joint Surgery, p. 1187.

Blumel, Johanna: "Eight Cases of Heriditary Bilateral Medial Tibial Torsion in Four Generations," Journal of Bone and Joint Surgery, October, 1957, Vol. 39-A, No. 5, p. 1198.

Bobath, Karel and Bobath, B.: "A Treatment of Cerebral Palsy Based on the Analysis of the Patient's Motive Behavior."

Brockman, E. P.: Congenital Clubfoot, London, Wright, 1930.

Bromberg, Murray: "The Role of the Ostibial Externum in Patho-Mechanical Disorders of the Foot," J.A.P.A., May, 1960, pp. 378.

Browne, Denis: Congenital Malformations Practitioner, England, 131:27-29, 1933.

Calmenson, Kermit: "Educational and Rehabilitative Approach to the Podiatrically Handicapped Child," J.A.P.A., February, 1962.

Cinzio, Joseph R.: Spastic Flatfoot, J. Nat. Assoc. Pod. 7,332, 1957.

Colonna, Paul C., Care of the Infant with Congenital Subluxation of the Hip. J.A.M.A., pp. 715-720, February 15, 1958.

Coventry, M. B. and Johnson, E. W., Jr.: Congenital Absence of the Fibula, Journal Bone & Joint Surg., 34-A, 941, 1952.

Crane, Lawrence: "Femoral Torsion and Its Relationship to Toeing-In and Toeing-Out," Journal of Bone and Joint Surgery, Vol. 41-A, p. 421.

Dickson, Frank D.: Posture, Its Relation to Health. J. B. Lippincott Co., Philadelphia, 1930.

Dorland's Medical Dictionary—24th Edition, W. B. Saunders, Philadelphia, Pa. 1965.

Dunlap, K. and Shands, A. R.: "A New Method for Determination of Torsion of the Femur."

Egel, Paula F.: Technique of Treatment for the Cerebral Palsy Child, C. V. Mosby Co., St. Louis, Mo.

Freiberg, A. H.: Infraction of the Second Metatarsal Bone, Surg., Gynec. & Obst., 19:191, 1914.

Garceau, G. J.: Filum Terminale Syndrome, Journal Bone and Joint Surg., 35-A: 711, 1953.

Harris, R. I. and Beath, T.: Etiology of Peroneal Spastic Flatfoot," J. Bone and Joint Surgery, November, 1948, Vol. 30-B, pp. 624-634.

Harris, R. I. and Beath, T.: "Retrospect-Perineal Spastic Flatfoot (Rigid Valgus Foot), "Journal Bone and Joint Surgery, December, 1965, p. 1657.

Hart, Vernon L.: Congenital Dislocation of the Hip in the Newborn and in Early Postnatal Life. J.A.M.A. August 12, 1950, pp. 1299-1303.

Helfet, A. J.: New Way of Treating Flat Feet in Children, Lancet, February 11, 1956, pp. 262-264.

Hutter, Charles G., Jr. and Scott, Walter: "Tibial Torsion," Journal of Bone and Joint Surgery, Vol. 31-A, p. 511.

Johnson, E. W. and Spiegel, M. H.: Ambulation Problems in Very Young Children, J.A.M.A., March 11, 1961, pp. 858-863.

Katz, J. F.: Congenital Absence of the Sacrum and Coccyx, Journal Bone and Joint Surg., 35-A; 398, 1953.

Kite, J. H.: "Tibial Torsion," Journal Bone and Joint Surgery, 36-A; 511, 1954.

Kite, J. H.: "Congenital Metatarsus Varus," Journal Bone and Joint Surgery, 32-A; 500, 1950.

Kite, J. H.: "Some Suggestions on the Treatment of Club Foot By Casts," Journal of Bone and Joint Surgery, Vol. 45-A, No. 2, March 1963, p. 406-412.

Knight, R. A.: "Developmental Deformities of the Lower Extremities," Journal Bone and Joint Surgery, Vol. 36-A: 521, 1954.

Koehler, Alban: Roentgenology, ed. 2, London, Baltiere, Tindall and Cox, 1935.

Krantz, Milton H.: Treating Childhood Gait Problems of the Denis Browne Toe, J.A.P.A., May 1960, p. 375.

Legg, A. T.: An Obscure Affection of the Hip Joint, Boston Med. and Surg. J., 162:202, 1910.

Lerner, Leonard H.: "Radiographic Evaluation of Calcaneal Apophysites," J.A.P.A., September, 1957, p. 451.

Lorenz, A.: Uber die Behandlung der Irrepibilen Angeborenen Huftuxationen und der Schenkelhalspseudoarthrosen.

Luck, J. F.: Bone and Joint Diseases, Springfield, Illinois, Thomas, 1950.

McCauley, John, Jr. Lusskin, Ralph, and Bromley, John: "Recurrence in Congenital Metatarsus Varsus," Journal of Bone and Joint Surgery, April, 1964, p. 525.

McKeever, Duncan Co.: "Interpretation and Treatment of Weight-Bearing Defects in Apparently Healthy Children," Vol. I, Clinical Orthopedics, J. B. Lippincott Co.

Meade, James C.: Juvenile Pes Plano Valgus, J.A.P.A., April, 1962, p. 475.

Milhoral, A. T.: Therapy in Muscular Dystrophy, Medical Annals, Dist. of Columbia; Jan. 1954; pp. 15-22.

Outland and Murphy: "Relation of Tarsal Anomalies to Spastic and Rigid Flat Feet," Clinical Orthopedics, Vol. I, J. B. Lippincott Co., 1953, p. 217-225.

Perlstein, M. A.: "Infantile Cerebral Palsy—Classification and Clinical Correlations," J.A.M.A., May 3, 1952, p. 30-34.

Phelps, W. H.: The Diagnosis and Treatment of Postural Defects, Baltiere, Tindall and Cox, London, 1932.

Powers, Dr. Margaret Hall: Chicago School System. Personal Communication.

Raney, Richard B. and Shands, Alfred R.: The Prevention of Deformity in Childhood. Kingsport Press, Kingsport, Tennessee.

Rhine, Irwin and Locke, Raymond K.: Osteochondrosis of Secondary Epiphysis of Calcaneus. Journal A.O.A., May, 1952, p. 441-447.

Roberts, P. W.: The Influence of the Os Calcis on the Production and Correction of Valgus Deformities of the Foot," Amer. Jour. Orthop. Surgery, December, 1916, XIV, Boston, pp. 720-725.

Rosen, H. and Sandrich, H.: Measurement of Tibio-Fibular Torsion, Journal Bone & Joint Surgery, Vol. 37-A, p. 847.

Ryder, Charles T. and Crane, Lawrence: "Measuring Femoral Anteversion: The Problem and Method," Journal Bone and Joint Surg., Vol. 35-A: 321-328, 1953.

Scheimer, Oscar M.: "The Chiropedical Management of Infantile Metatarsus Varus," J.A.P.A., December, 1947, p. 435.

Shands, A. R.: "Care and Treatment of Crippled Children in the U.S.," Journal of Bone and Joint Surgery, January, 1953.

Swanson, Alfred B.: "Rotational Deformities of the Lower Extremity in Children and Their Clinical Significance."

Thomsen, J. E. M.: "Treatment of Congenital Flat-foot," Journal Bone and Joint Surgery, Vol. 28:787-790, 1946.

Wartenberg, R.: "Plantar Reflex," The Examination of Reflexes, Year Book Publishers, Chicago, 1945.

Watson, Ernest H. and Lowrey, George H.: Growth and Development of Children, Year Book Publishers, Chicago, 1951.

Waugh, W.: The Ossification and Vascularization of the Tarsal Navicular and Their Relation to Kohler's Disease, Journal Bone and Joint Surg., 40-B: 765, 1958.

ILLUSTRATIONS